GOD BLESS AMERICA!

Dr. Wallach's Nutritional, Health and Survival Epiphany!

GOD BLESS AMERICA!

Dr. Wallach's Nutritional, Health and Survival Epiphany!

Dr J. D. Wallach, BS, DVM, ND & Dr Ma Lan, MD, MS, LAc

Wellness Publications, L.L.C.

Library of Congress Cataloging in Publications Data:
Wallach, J.D. and Lan, Ma

GOD BLESS AMERICA!
    Bibliography
    Includes index
    1. Longevity 2. Medical Dogmas 3. Diets 4. Centenarians
    5. Nutrition 6. Self defense 7. Biological warfare 8. chemi-
    cal warfare 9. Longevity recipes 10. Soil depletion 11. Food
    nutrient depletion 12: Pica 13. Financial planning for 100
    year olds. 14. Home defense. 15. Nuclear, biological and
    chemical attacks and defense

GOD BLESS AMERICA!
First Edition, January 2002
Second Edition, January 2013

Printed and published by Wellness Publications, L.L.C.
P.O. Box 1222, Bonita, California 91902.
www.drjwallach.com
1 – 800 – 755 – 4656 USA and Canada
1 – 619 – 420 – 2435 local and international

Table of Contents

ABOUT THE AUTHORS

Joel D. Wallach, BS, DVM, ND

Dr. Wallach has been involved in biomedical research and clinical medicine for more than 44 years. He received his B.S. degree (agriculture) from the University of Missouri with a major in animal husbandry (nutrition) and a minor in field crops and soils; a D.V.M. (veterinarian) from the University of Missouri; a three year post doctoral Ames, Iowa, Natal Parks Board, Umfolozi and Hluehluwe Game Parks, Republic of South Africa, The Center for the Biology of Natural Systems, Washington University, the St. Louis Zoological Gardens, the Chicago Zoological Gardens (Brookfield Zoo), the Yerkes Regional Primate Research Center, Emory University, Atlanta, Georgia, the National College of Naturopathic Medicine, Portland, Oregon, Harbin Medical University, Harbin, Hei Long Jiang and the Shanghai Medical University, People's Republic of China.

He was a member of NIH site visit teams for facilities using exotic animal models for the study of human disease for four years and was a member of the 1968 National Science Foundation ad hoc committee that authored the 1968 Animal Welfare Act (humane housing, nutrition and care of laboratory and captive exotic species); and a Consulting Professor of Medicine, Harbin Medical University, Harbin, Hei Long Jiang, People's Republic of China.

Dr. Wallach attained the rank of Lieutenant Colonel in the Missouri Air National Guard (131st Tactical Hospital), known as "Lindberg's own," and the Alaskan Air Reserves with responsibilities in public health and prevention and clean up of nuclear, biological and chemical attacks in North America and Europe.

Dr. Wallach was the recipient of the Wooster Beach Gold Medal Award for a significant breakthrough in the basic understanding of the cause and pathophysiology of Cystic Fibrosis---the Wooster Beech gold medal was awarded by the Association of Eclectic Physicians. Dr. Wallach was nominated for the Nobel

Prize in Medicine in 1991 by the Association of Eclectic Physicians for his work in the understanding of the genesis and pathophysiology of cystic fibrosis.

Dr.Wallach has appeared frequently on local and national network television (including a special on cystic fibrosis with ABC's 20/20), regional and national talk radio programs as an expert on trace mineral and rare earth deficiency diseases. Dr.Wallach is also the host of his own syndicated talk show radio programs (Let's Play Doctor and Dead Doctors Don't Lie). Because of his freewheeling style of humor and ability to quickly zero in on the basic truth in health problems and medical politics he is widely known as the "Rush Limbaugh" of alternative health.

Ma Lan MD, MS, Lac

Dr. Ma Lan was educated in the People's Republic of China. Dr. Ma Lan received her MD from the Beijing Medical University, took her residency at the People's Hospital, Beijing and was a staff surgeon at the Canton Air Force Hospital, she received her MS (Master of Science) in transplantation immunology from Zhongshan Medical University, Canton, People's Republic of China; as with all Chinese doctors, Dr. Ma Lan was trained in Traditional Chinese Medicine (i.e.- acupuncture, herbs, manipulation, food medicine, massage and hydrotherapy) prior to entering the Western-style medical school.

Dr. Ma Lan's research credits include being an exchange scholar at Harvard School of Medicine, Boston, MA; a research fellow in laser microsurgery at St. Joseph Hospital, Houston, TX; the Department of Orthopedic Microsurgery at the Medical College of Wisconsin, Milwaukee, WI and the Department of Pharmacology at the University of California, San Diego, CA. Dr. Ma Lan has 10 peer review publications to her credit in the fields of transplant immunology and laser vascular microsurgery. Dr. Ma Lan attained the rank of lieutenant in the Chinese Air Force with primary responsibilities as a general surgeon in the Canton Air Force Hospital, PRC.

Dr. J.D. Wallach and Dr. Ma Lan joint book & booklet publications

Let's Play Doctor 1989

RARE EARTHS: forbidden cures 1994

Dead Doctors Don't Lie! 1997

Let's Play Herbal Doctor 2000

Biological and Chemical Attacks on America 2001 (16 pg)

INTRODUCTION

Medical doctors have long discounted the concept that individuals could actively and significantly increase their life span beyond 120 years and that 120 year olds were one in six billion – today, learned gerantologists and geneticists agree that 120 to 150 years of age is not only a reasonable expectation but well within the average American's genetic capability of achieving through simple dietary and supplement programs – in fact many experts believe that 200 or more is a reasonable expectation if one does everything right!

GOD BLESS AMERICA! is a collection of seemingly unrelated pieces of understanding necessary to grasp the full concept of what needs to be done to ensure making it to a healthful life at 200 years of age – to be sure these pieces of the health and longevity puzzle have never been aligned, connected and completed before – this is Dr. Wallach's EPIPHANY!

Longevity research projects that there will be up to 5 million Americans over the age of 100 by the year 2050 and that many Americans will achieve ages of over 200 years if they consciously employ all known health, nutrition and supplement information already available. Nutrition research goes on to demonstrate that for every dollar spent for supplements under the age of 50 will save you three dollars in health care over the age of 50!

Most people forget, that to live comfortably as a 100 year old, you will need to avoid the land mines, supplement with all 90 essential nutrients and establish cash flow and passive incomes that could, if necessary carry you to 120, 140 and even to 200 years of age. If you start developing your passive cash flow resources the moment you finish this book you will be part of a small elite group – centenarians with enough health and money to live well.

Many medical groups have attacked Dr. Wallach personally in the print media to try to demonize him and to discredit him (i.e.-

no way he could do that many autopsies, anybody can be nominated for the Nobel Prize, he is in his sixties, balding and too
round in the middle, his claim that doctors don't live as long as the
average American is false, he is a bizarre caricature of a quack,
etc.), yet none have attacked his health and longevity conclusions
or nutritional advice! When you can't attack the science, attack
the messenger personally is their historical and shameful M.O.

I have tried many times to debate doctors on radio, television
and in public forums with the agreement that they would have to
sign a contract that says they must debate the issues and the science and not attack me personally, but doctors will always refuse
– if they can't attack me personally they just won't participate in
a debate of the health issues and the value of nutritional supplement programs because they know that Dr. Wallach's EPIPHANY
is the truth.

There are no laws that require doctors to cure people even
when there are cures available. There are no laws that require doctors to teach people how to prevent disease even when disease
preventions are available. From the moment a doctor starts up a
new practice his or her sole focus is to "build" a practice, to get
as many people as possible on long-term treatment, therapy and
prescription pharmaceutical programs. A medical practice that
has no ongoing patient visits, because they have all been cured, is
of no value when it comes time to get a loan, estimate net worth
or sell the practice. A medical practice with 10,000 active patient
files with an average visit rate of four visits per year per patient
is worth millions!

GOD BLESS AMERICA! is designed to compile all of the known
human longevity information, health, nutrition, self-defense and
financial secrets that have been widely proven over time to be
useful for one or more cultures – the proof is in the pudding.

Dr. J.D. Wallach and Dr. Ma Lan

Acknowledgements and Disclaimers

We gratefully acknowledge the editing, help and council of Steve Wallach, Dr. Gerhardt Schrauzer, Phyllis Wright, Craig Walcott, Vince Marasigan, Tina Danielsen and Bay Port Press. We gratefully acknowledge the Nature's Whey recipes provided by Les Lyons.

None of what is written in this book is approved or sanctioned for humans by the FDA, HHS, FTC, ATF, SEC, SEC (this is not a typo), CDC, DOD, FBI, CIA, FAA, FCC, KGB, IRS, BTF, BLM, DEA, USDA, GAO, OMB, NASA, PETA, NAFTA, NCAA, VA, NATO, SEATO, OAS, EU, FICA, FDIC, FSLIC, HUD, USPS, PSTA, PTA, UN or the Red Cross. The contents of this book have not been reviewed with Generally Accepted Accounting Principals by the accounting firm of Arthur Anderson.

Chapter 1

Behold the awakening of a sleeping giant

"Be prepared!"

—Motto
Boy Scouts of America

According to the Constitution of the United States, the purpose of the federal government is to protect Americans from enemies foreign and domestic – to that end our government has been an abysmal failure in the late 20th and early 21st centuries. After the time of Teddy Roosevelt (talk softly and carry a big stick), U.S. Senators and U.S. Representatives (at the urging of the pharmaceutical and medical industries) have spent more time, energy and tax money harassing alternative thought (Waco, Ruby Ridge), alternative health care professionals and the producers of vitamin, mineral and herbal supplements and crushing private businesses simply because they were successful (i.e.- Microsoft, etc.) than they have in protecting Americans (i.e.– the WTC 1993 bombing, the marines in Lebanon, the Oklahoma City federal building, the U.S. special forces in Somalia, U.S. embassies in Nairobi, Kenya, East Africa, the USS Cole in Yemen, the 9/11 WTC twin towers attack, the Pentagon attack and the post 9/11 anthrax bio-terror attacks).

In each instance our domestic and foreign intelligence services failed to detect the terrorist's sinister activities and their actual crime before their evil deeds were done and we were left with the job of cleaning up the tangles of steel and bodies and chasing and catching criminals and terrorists on a global theater.

There are no real emergencies when one is prepared. The reason that the Y2K "Millennium Bug" passed into the year 2000 with a whimper, was not because there was no real danger for disruption of our computer systems, our delivery systems, health services, police services, firefighting services, food and water supplies but rather everyone (every individual, corporation and every city, county, state and federal agency) in America was aware, became paranoid and prepared – Y2K? Ho-hum!

There were actual and potential disruptions of utility services that occurred on January 1, 2000, however, because of the general state of American preparedness there was nothing really newsworthy that appeared in the national TV or print media. Wasn't it better to be over prepared than under prepared?

The 9/11 WTC twin towers, the Pentagon attacks of September 11, 2001 and the anthrax biological attacks that followed are symptoms of the federal government's impotence and continued failure to "stay ahead of the curve" on many fronts; and like the Y2K challenge individual Americans and the private business sector are going to have to take the initiative, take a stand, educate themselves and the public and be prepared for a total collapse of private and government services including health care should additional attacks take place. We are fighting a two-front war – incompetence and misdirected beaureaucratic energy and resources on the home front (CIA, FBI and CDC) and a do or die war against every now emboldened terrorist group in and outside of America.

The advantage our patients and associates have had over the years is the fact that both Dr. Ma Lan and myself have spent many years in the military dealing with military and civilian mass disaster scenarios; I am a veterinarian as well as a physician and can translate the scientific research and medical language of both animals and humans to useful information. Hundreds of billions of dollars of animal nutritional research have been accumulated since the1930s when purified laboratory diets were first conceived. Medical doctors, the government and the private pharmaceutical industries controlled by doctors accept pharmaceutical studies performed in animals because they get paid kickbacks or given perks to believe, yet do not foster animal studies for basic nutritional research - not because the animal nutritional studies lack truth or because of a lack of scientific validity but rather for arrogant turf battles and overt money grabbing and price gouging by the medical community and pharmaceutical empires.

The advantage that Dr. Ma Lan and I have had over the years as physicians is a unique collection of background experiences and training beginning in the livestock industry and farming, agricultural school, veterinary school, postdoctoral fellowship in comparative medicine and comparative pathology, primary care physician (ND), medical doctor (MD), general surgery, microsurgery, Chinese traditional medicine, herbal medicine, clinical nutritional medicine, military emergencies and public health with over 75 years of combined biomedical and clinical research in animals and humans.

I have performed, reviewed and analyzed more than 17,500 autopsies in over 454 species of animals and 3,000 human beings. These background experiences have allowed Dr. Ma Lan and myself to come to the unimpeachable truth that every animal and every human being that dies of natural causes dies of a nutritional deficiency disease – Dr. WALLACH'S NUTRITIONAL EPIPHANY!

That little sentence "you can get every thing you need from the basic four food groups" has killed more Americans than all of the wars, terrorist attacks and muggings put together in the 220 years we have been a nation. You cannot get everything you nutritionally need from the four basic food groups or by following the USDA's seven food group pyramid, because grains, fruit, nuts and vegetables cannot manufacture minerals, and nutritional minerals are not found in a uniform blanket over the crust of the Earth. Where there were no minerals in the soil, there are still no minerals in the soil. Where there were once veins of nutritional minerals in the soil those veins are now depleted. You must supplement with all 90 essential nutrients, especially the 60 essential minerals to be able to fulfill your genetic potential for longevity and warrantee maximum lifespan and healthy longevity.

Eating well and believing and hoping that all 90 essential nutrients are in your meals because we are Americans is giving yourself into slavery with the medical system and medical doctors the slave masters without even a whimper of complaint or resistance – whatever happened to "Give me liberty or give me death!"

The Earth's atmosphere and its oxygen content is the same the world over, the molecular make-up of unpolluted water is the same the world over, but the soil we grow our food in is different in its mineral content from row to row, field to field, county to county, state to state, country to country and continent to continent. The big health and life-threatening variable in our environment is not pollution, but rather the food value or lack of food value of the soil we grow our food in.

Grains, vegetables, fruit and nuts can in fact use the carbon dioxide from the air, the sun's energy and a process known as photosynthesis to manufacture beta carotene, vitamins A, B complex, vitamin C, vitamin E, vitamin K, vitamin D, amino acids and fatty acids - plants however, can't manufacture nutritional minerals – if they aren't in the soil they aren't in our food!

Plants depend on the soil as their sole source of minerals. Unfortunately, the 60 essential minerals, known to be required for animal and human health, do not occur in a uniform blanket cloaking the crust of the Earth. Rather, the 60 essential minerals occur randomly in the soil as veins, like veins of gold or silver or like chocolate in chocolate ripple ice cream.

It is this vast variation in soil mineral content that produces the wide disparity that exists in the average age from country to country – 81.2 in Okinawa and 25.9 in Sierra Leone. The average

age variation from country to country is not due to the lack of money, the lack of western-style medical care or to a lousy throw of the genetic dice but rather the "haves and have-nots" of nutritional mineral resources in the soil.

The test of a classical EPIPHANY is to be able to reverse engineer the profound observation and use the new and more complete truth to significantly better mankind, create a new science, or initiate an industrial, scientific or cultural revolution, however, despite our best efforts over our combined 75 years of professional effort, medical dogma, ego and turf protection behavior by medical doctors has discounted and viciously attacked the EPIPHANY.

The audio tape Dead Doctors Don't Lie illustrated the fact that family doctors didn't live as long as the average American back in 1994 - an original small study based on 44 obituaries collected from the January 20, 1992 issue of JAMA showed the average family doctor in America lived to an average age of 57.6 years. The hue and cry from the medical trade regarding the reporting of their short life span was vicious and deafening.

A larger 1999 more recent study on more than 900 doctors published in the Archives of Otolaryngology, Head and Neck Surgery reported that family practitioners in America only lived to be an average of 56 years, redeeming my initial study - hardly a testimony to the claim that "doctor knows best!"

Dr. Wallach's EPIPHANY on health and longevity was first presented to the general public in 1978 and to our great joy the American public was ready to leave the old medical dogmas and lies behind and move forward to a more universal health truth already proven at great expense in the animal industry. Since 1978 millions of Americans and untold numbers of Canadians, Europeans and Asians have utilized the truths gained from Dr. Wallach's EPIPHANY to better their lives, gain better health and move towards fulfilling their genetic potential for longevity.

Like the minutemen on the American frontier, each of us will have to provide our own first line of defense against cunning and vicious enemies foreign and domestic; we will have to be our own lookouts, our own defenders of our families and community, our own doctors and our own providers of utilities, public health, hygiene and the funding of our post-100 year life style.

Three hundred million Americans cannot depend on federal, state, county or city governments to provide for our every human need as there is not the community will or enough money in the world to support such a project (the communists and socialists have tried such a plan and have failed over and over again) – we must be vigilant, we must be activists, we must be independent and we must be the new minutemen!

Many tens of millions who have listened to the Dead Doctors Don't Lie audio tape, read the book Dead Doctors Don't Lie, listened to our syndicated radio programs or attended Dr. Wallach's free Dead Doctors Don't Lie health lectures have asked for more details, specific meals and recipes, supplement programs, personal safety dealing with disruption of public utilities, how to defend against nuclear, biological and chemical attacks, how to finance being a centenarian and for simple recipes that would give life to the EPIPHANY for the average American – *GOD BLESS AMERICA!* is our answer to those requests.

GOD BLESS AMERICA! And God Bless Our Centenarians!

Chapter 2

Food Fight!

"Those who now advocate eating natural foods as the only source of vitamins and minerals live in a dream world of yesterday. What was yesterday's law is today's folly. It really doesn't matter how well you balance your meals, or if you're a meat eater, vegetarian or a raw-foodist, you still run the risk of malnutrition if you try to get all your vitamins and minerals exclusively from the foods you eat."

—Pavo Airola, PhD
The Airola Diet and Cook Book

There are many diets and diet gurus competing for armies of zealous followers, each testifying as to the benefits and singular perfection of vision and scientific approach of their diet and their "way of life." The test of the current "truth" always comes with the test of time - as time is no respecter of theory or prophet - truth like cream always rises to the top.

Diets and food fads are concocted and promoted for weight loss, weight control, beauty, spiritual enlightenment, diagnosis, detoxification, "cleansing," energy, health, cures for chronic disease, fertility, sexual prowess, strength, speed, stamina and longevity.

Some diets have been raised to the level of medical dogma (i.e.- four food groups, seven-food group pyramid, Mediterranean diet, etc.) and have become the constant blind dogma and ignorant mantra of medical doctors, dieticians and self anointed food experts, yet the life spans of those cultures and individuals who follow the teachings of the four food groups, the seven food group pyramid and the Mediterranean diet continues to drop - the

Italians from 75.5 in 1990 to 72.7 in 2000, Americans plummeted from an average life span of 75 years and ranking 17th in the world for longevity in 1990 to an average life span of 70 years and 24th in longevity in 2000 when compared with the top 32 First World countries.

The Japanese maintained their status as the longest-lived industrial culture over the same 10-year period at 79.1 years in 1990 to 75 years in 2000, yet western doctors claim the Japanese do everything wrong. They smoke heavily, they fry or stir fry almost everything they eat including rice, vegetables and animal protein, they eat raw fish with worms in them (sushi), they eat 12 grams of salt each day (three times that recommended by American doctors) and we dropped two atomic bombs on them – the Japanese have soaked up more radiation per person than any other culture on earth, yet the Japanese live more than four years longer than the average American and have 85% less breast, prostate and colon cancer and cardiovascular disease rates we do! HELLO – there is a message here!

Eighty five percent of all Americans dutifully march to a medical doctor each year for their annual physical, respect their doctor and for the most part make every effort to follow their doctors advice – yet, our average American life span has remained about 75, give or take a few years for the last 50 years and our world ranking in longevity dropped from 17th to 24th.

The entire world spent $2.7 trillion for health care in 1998, and of that mind-boggling medical cost, the United States spent $1.5 trillion - more than half! Americans have access to medical technology that is the envy of the entire world, yet despite having the most expensive and the most technologically advanced health care system in the world (Americans spend more than half of the entire world's total expenditure for health care) our average life span remains 75 and we currently rank 24th in the world for longevity.

The three top G-7 countries ranked behind the U.S. (the richest and most technologically advanced countries in the world) that try to mimic the medical philosophy and technology of the U.S. don't fare very well when it comes to quality of health care according to the WHO: 1) UK – 18th; 2) Germany – 25th; 3) Canada – 30th; 4) U.S. – 37th.

All of these statistics indicate that we are on the wrong train, we are headed in the wrong direction and that we are paying for first class tickets and winding up riding in the caboose! Americans wouldn't tolerate such service from Amtrak – why do we tolerate such poor service from medical doctors?

A review and critique of some of the more current and historically important and popular diets is of value as there are pieces of some diets that are still of use, some should be consciously avoided and others that have simply died because the basic theory was faulty, impractical or incomplete.

The low fat/low cholesterol diets promoted for the last 50 years by orthodox and alternative health experts have failed to increase the nations average lifespan or maximum lifespan. In fact, the advent of low animal fat diets and high plant oil intakes have paralleled a reduction in America's IQ level and the sudden appearance of a number of new diseases (physician caused fat and cholesterol deficiency diseases) including acquired seizure disorders, fibromyalgia, Alzheimer's disease, and the increase in rates of long known diseases including depression, asthma, cancer and adult onset type II diabetes and the most telling statistic of all – a drop from 17th in the world ranking for longevity to 24th (there are now 23 other countries whose peoples live longer than Americans).

When dietary and total blood cholesterol levels were lowered by diet, exercise and statin drugs nothing significant happened in the positive column for Americans. The discovery of "good HDL" and "bad LDL" cholesterol and the attainment of their proper blood ratio produced little or no longevity benefit for Americans. In fact there is not a single disease caused by elevated blood cholesterol or elevated blood triglycerides. Elevated blood cholesterol (above 270) and elevated triglycerides (above 75) are in fact warning signals not unlike a fever. One gets a fever with viral, bacterial and parasite infections, cancer, liver disease, bone fractures and teething.

One can get elevated blood cholesterol and elevated blood triglycerides when they have hypothyroidism (low functioning thyroid), diabetes, deficiencies of niacin (vitamin B3), chromium, vanadium, the essential fatty acids and liver disease, however elevated blood cholesterol and blood triglycerides in of themselves do not cause disease.

Can you ever remember your veterinarian getting excited about your dog's, cat's, fish, bird's or livestock's blood cholesterol or triglycerides – absolutely not! We've known for 75 years in the animal industry that elevated blood cholesterol or triglycerides are not bogeymen, they do not cause a single disease and just lowering cholesterol and triglycerides in of themselves do not reduce risk for or cure any disease.

Medical doctors on the cutting edge of cardiovascular disease research have all but given up on cholesterol and triglycerides and the ratios of good (HDL) and bad (LDL) cholesterol as the cause of cardiovascular disease. Frustrated doctors turned to elevated blood homocystine levels, which is a simple biochemical marker for a folic acid deficiency. Having quickly abandoned the homocystine theory, cardiologist then blamed a simple oral bacterium as the cause of arteriosclerotic cardiovascular disease. Currently a lutien (a flavonoid found in egg yolk and green vegetables) and magnesium deficiencies seem a most likely candidates as the cause of calcium (metastatic calcification) and fatty deposits in our arteries.

In fact the more eggs you eat the less likely you are to develop coronary artery disease and stroke; and in fact the lower your blood cholesterol gets the more likely you are to get stroke, intracranial hemorrhage, chronic obstructive pulmonary disease and liver cancer by as much as 200 to 300 percent.

One report in March 1991 issue of the New England Journal of Medicine highlighted an 88-year old man who ate 25 eggs per day and had normal cholesterol levels. A modern review of the habits of centenarians published in the journal Scientific American September 2000, showed that they pay no attention to dietary or blood cholesterol levels and that they often eat a hearty egg laden breakfast every morning, smoke and don't exercise.

Despite the 50 year hysteria over cholesterol, despite the massive societal shift to a low cholesterol consumption and drug induced reductions in blood cholesterol levels Americans dropped from 17th in longevity out of the top 32 industrialized nations in 1990 to 24th in longevity in the year 2000 – a seven slot drop despite low and no cholesterol foods, more statin drugs to lower cholesterol, more bypass surgery, more stints and more heart transplants, more after care. It is quite obvious that we haven't gotten the message or the bang for our buck when it comes to health and longevity by simply lowering cholesterol.

Vegetarianism means different things to different people. To most, giving up feed lot fattened red meat means one is a vegetarian, yet most "vegetarians" will eat range reared poultry, eggs, seafood, dairy, range fed or organically grown beef and lamb and wild game. These hybrid "vegetarian" or omnivore type diets when supplemented properly with a full compliment of all 90 essential nutrients can be tweaked into the perfect human diet.

The vegan diet is perhaps the most cruel of all diets because the prophets of veganism implore recruits to join their numbers for spiritual and health reasons, yet there are no flourishing colonies of vegans with robust middle-aged people, giggling children skipping around or that have a large percentages of centenarians to show off as the rewards of the vegan lifestyle. Some of the sickest people (both emotionally and physically) you will ever meet are vegans. There has never been a vegan who has lived to be 100 years of age!

Most vegans are told and believe they are following the correct dietary path, because they can (with considerable effort) get a complete amino acid spectrum by simply mixing grains and legumes, however, the vegan's concern for and their zeal to obtain the other 78 essential nutrients is shallow or non-existent.

There are 90 essential nutrients and betting one's health, fertility and longevity or worse yet the health and longevity of one's children on what might be or might not be in one's seven-grain bread is simply throwing one's life away. All strict vegans will suffer from multiple deficiencies of minerals (i.e.- calcium, sulfur, copper, zinc, iron, selenium, chromium, vanadium, iodine, lithium, etc.), vitamin B12 and cholesterol.

As a result of their restricted and commonly un-supplemented diets, vegans tend to be "wigged out," have anxiety attacks, panic attacks, depression, bipolar disease, chemical imbalances, chronic fatigue syndrome, fibromyalgia, osteoporosis, arthritis, periodontal disease, infertility, hypoglycemia, hyperinsulinemia (narcolepsy) and a host of other chronic diseases including diabetes, lupus and Alzheimer's disease.

Vegans would have their followers believe that the Chinese and other oriental cultures are vegetarians - nothing is further from the truth. The Chinese eat four to six servings of animal protein per meal including fish, squid, octopus, shrimp, shellfish, poultry, pigeons, duck, chicken eggs, duck eggs, quail eggs, pork, beef, deer, goat, lamb, rabbit, amphibians, snakes, snails, dog, cat and historically in times of great famine they ate human flesh.

Traditionally the Chinese do not eat dairy products, however, they do boil bones of all animals in vinegar and drink and eat the bone soup as their major source of calcium.

There has never been a single vegan who became a vegan after weaning off of their mother's breast milk and remained a vegan throughout life who has lived to be a hundred. Proper intense supplementation can make up for most of the nutritional shortcomings of a vegan diet, however, novices are prevented from vigorously supplementing by misguided and overzealous peer and prophet pressure. One such victim was the late international vegan spokesperson Linda McCartney (wife of Beatle Paul McCartney) who died of breast cancer at age 54.

Blood type based diets have come and gone and again come

and gone. Choosing your diet based on your blood type was an original thought of Dr. William Kelly, a dentist from Texas who was diagnosed with terminal pancreatic cancer in the 1960s. Kelly believed that he could individualize his own and other cancer patient's diet program based on their blood type – 40 years later he is still alive and kicking.

This "eat right for your blood type" concept has been abandoned by most alternative cancer hospitals because without correct supplementation and constant monitoring it turns out to be a starvation diet for people with blood types A, B, AB and O. In recent years the "eat right for your blood type" diet has briefly been popularized again.

The current authors and proponents of the "eat right for your blood type" diet suggest the reason why the "eat for your blood type" diet doesn't work for everyone is that there are blood subgroups (i.e.- Rh factors, genetic factors, etc.) that have to be factored into the equation for the diet to be followed correctly and to gain the maximum benefit.

Reduced calorie diets or "undernutrition without malnutrition" have been looked at in one-celled animals, spiders, mice, rats, fish and monkeys since Clive Mckay's restricted calorie rat diets in the 1930s extended rats life spans as much as double that of normally fed rats; and when supplemented properly undernutrition without malnutrition diets can increase healthfulness and increase life-spans by as much as 10% to 100%.

The phrase "without malnutrition" is double-speak code by antagonist to supplementation for the serious supplementation of vitamins, major minerals, trace minerals and rare earths necessary for the restricted calorie diet to be safe and effective. Without increasing the concentration of nutritional minerals per carbohydrate calorie a reduced calorie diet will cause an increased rate of appearance of chronic degenerative diseases and increased death rate in young immature laboratory animals and humans as well as older individuals.

Recent attempts to put humans on reduced calorie diets (less than 1,500 calories per day) without serious attention to the supplement part of the equation resulted in serious health problems. The Biosphere II low calorie adventure was a failure. Many seniors who restrict calories without increasing the concentration of minerals per carbohydrate calorie exhaust their energy and nutrient reserves, which often times results in the appearance of new diseases, accelerated aging and early death.

Variations of the original Clive McKay reduced calorie diet in rats include Roy Walford's "The 120 Year Diet," which reduces total calories to 1200 per day but keeps 60 % of calories from carbohydrate (a great way to produce fatigue and get fat); the Barry Sears' "Zone Diet" which reduces the ratio of carbohydrate calories to 20% of total calories; the Atkin's Diet which touts a low carbohydrate and high protein diet and the Dr. Wallach's Seefood Diet that all but eliminates carbohydrate calories (there are no nutritional requirements for carbohydrate) and significantly ramps up supplemental major mineral, trace mineral and rare earth intakes.

The macrobiotic diet, a.k.a. "The brown rice diet," which was created in Germany in the 1700s, was originally designed to be a short term "cleansing" diet ranging in duration from one week to one month. The original macrobiotic cleansing diet was a diet restricted to brown rice, fruit and vegetables - the original macrobiotic diet was never designed to be a lifelong practice. The main theme of the macrobiotic diet was to give up wheat, dairy and meat. There is no magic to be found in a brown rice or the macrobiotic diet, but the fact that wheat has been eliminated from one's diet helps many people who have sub-clinical or full blown celiac disease as a result of intestinal lining repair and improved absorption of macronutrients and micronutrients.

People who adhered strictly to the original macrobiotic diet for long periods of time as a cancer prevention program developed severe energy reserve depletion, protein deficiency and micronutrient deficiencies (i.e.- vitamins, major minerals and trace minerals). Tragically the wife of Micshio Kuhci, the 1970's

Japanese macrobiotic diet guru, died in 2001 at the age of 78 from breast cancer. The modern version of the macrobiotic diet has added fish as a more complete protein source. The macrobiotic diet, which today simulates the coastal Japanese or Okinawan diet, even without supplementation can benefit many over the short haul and increase the number of people reaching the average age of 75 years of age, but the macrobiotic diet will not add centenarians to the charts without adding a heavy and complete mineral supplementation program to it.

The traditional Okinawa diet is unique in the Japanese Empire in that it is a modest carbohydrate, moderate calorie, high protein and high mineral cuisine. The heavy consumption of fish and shellfish and the consumption of heavily mineralized sea vegetables are credited with the legendary Okinawa longevity. Interestingly enough Okinawans have the longest average lifespan of any culture at 81.2, yet they do not have an extraordinary number of centenarians at 34/100,000.

The much lauded Okinawan longevity was only recorded after the introduction of many western type foods to their diet following World War II; the current generation of Okinawans have all but given up the traditional Okinawan diet and as a result are not showing the same health and longevity benefits exhibited by the "old ones".

The paeleolithic diet or raw food diet actually increases the risk of mineral deficiency diseases. The phytate content of high fiber raw vegetables, whole grains and bran binds onto nutritional minerals and makes them unavailable for efficient absorption. The "Ice Man" or Otzie, whose frozen 5,000 year-old body was found in the Italian Alps was only 40 years old when he died (killed by an arrow wound in the back), yet he was riddled with arthritis of the hips, shoulder and ribs and arteriosclerosis of the aorta, coronary and iliac arteries. The value of an un-supplemented paeleolithic diet (if there was one) is that it is a very low carbohydrate diet.

The "carb-up" diet of the athlete of the 80's and 90's was an attempt to pack quick energy glycogen (animal starch) into the liver, skeletal and cardiac muscle cells the night before an event. This carbohydrate for energy approach to cellular energy was great for short and middle distance runners, but an abysmal failure for long distance runners and other high output four quarter sports or the third quarter athletes who would "hit the wall" or run out of steam (hypoglycemia) somewhere around the halfway mark or the third quarter.

It is now well established that a high animal fat intake (T-bone steak) the night before an extended output athletic event was more likely to produce the sustained energy source and reserves required for stamina than a pasta dinner.

Juicing and concocting multi-fruit and vegetable smoothies is one of the greatest ways I know of to get fresh and natural sources of beta carotene, lycopenes, lutiens, vitamin C, folic acid, some of the B-complex vitamins (certainly not vitamin B12), however, juicing will not provide a warranteed spectrum of all 60 essential minerals or sufficient amounts of each. After seven years of being associated with alternative cancer hospitals we can say with great accuracy that almost all patients (other than the Amish) were on some form of vegetarian and/or juicing programs long before they were diagnosed with cancer.

The USDA's seven-food group pyramid has been a failure right out of the chute! The same people who express dismay at the fattening of American children put six to 11 servings of carbohydrates as the base and flagship feature of the seven food pyramid! The seven-food group pyramid was designed for high-energy output athletes who can burn 5,000 calories per day, not for the average grade school student and the data entry guy.

If you want to make pigs fat give them carbohydrate! If you want to make cattle fat give them carbohydrate! If you want to make Americans fat give them the seven-food group pyramid!

The omnivore diet covers all kinds of mixed ethnic diet types diets that include various combinations of eggs, fish, poultry, red meat as well as grains, vegetables, nuts, fruit and exotic spices; these broad spectrum ethnic diets are the most practical of the dietary practices that contain the maximum levels of nutrition from non-supplemented food combinations. The old admonition to consume a variety of food in one's diet increased the chances of blundering into a greater variety of essential nutrients. And by simple observation over time rather than a scientific study, the omnivore diet showed the most universal success. The Okinawan version of variety is to make sure that there are foods of five different colors in each meal.

The carnivore or high meat diets consumed by the traditional Eskimo societies above the Arctic Circle are up to 98% red meat and blubber (i.e.- whale meat, whale blubber, walrus meat, walrus blubber, seal meat, seal blubber, bear meat, bear fat, etc.), their blood cholesterol levels range from 250 to 350 and yet they are legendary for having significantly lower rates of cardiovascular disease than black, white and Hispanic individuals in the "lower 48" who follow their doctors' advice and lower their intake of animal protein and animal fats.

The Eskimo's consumption of salmon and other cold-water fish provide rich sources of the Omega-3 essential fatty acids and reduce the risk of abnormally sticky platelets. The regular consumption of animal liver assures the Eskimo of an optimal intake of copper, selenium, rare earths, vitamin A, vitamin C, vitamin D and vitamin B12 thus significantly reducing the risk of aneurysms and cardiomyopathy heart disease.

Some bands of Eskimo eat animal bones and eliminate calcium deficiency diseases such as osteoporosis, arthritis and hypertension; other bands do not eat animal bone and develop arthritis, periodontal disease and osteoporosis.

The Mormon and the Seventh Day Adventist health laws and diets have long been known to statistically add up to10 additional years above the American average of 75 up to 85.5. Simply put, the Mormon and Seventh Day Adventist diet allows for consumption of most things in moderation but avoids pork (therefore a lot of fried food), caffeine, alcohol and smoking. It appears that the simple act of giving up just a few "bad things" can add as many as 10 additional good years to the average individuals lifespan (85.5) but doesn't extend the maximum lifespan at all.

After 30 years of frustrating crusades trying to get vegans to eat fish and eggs and carnivores to eat more vegetables, we came to the realization that we could not change significant numbers of zealots from any dietary or nutritional camp or philosophy to the middle ground so we decided to find a universal concept that would be acceptable to all and at the same time accomplish the purpose of optimal individual nutrition that would get maximal numbers of people through the hoops necessary to fulfill their genetic potential for longevity (120 to 140 years).

At first, we tried to formulate and calculate dietary programs for each nutritional cult, sect, fad and concept, but quickly realized that by its very nature trying to provide optimal nutrition through un-supplemented diets to any and all groups was faulty and reckless. We realized we couldn't change truck drivers and farmers from eating steaks and chops to organically grown broccoli and tofu any more than we could convert cats to vegetarianism; and by the same token we couldn't change a dot-comer's passion for bran muffins, yogurt and expresso coffee to eggs soft scrambled in butter, breakfast steak and sliced tomatoes any more than we could convert horses to eating red meat; and lastly to try to get Americans to adopt a 1,200 to 1,800 calorie a day reduced-calorie diet would be as difficult as trying to get Americans to join the Russian Red Army.

Even if we had been successful in putting together a collection of such dietary programs, the wide spread education and marketing challenges of such programs necessary to get them to the "guy on the streets" was an economic horror and an energy sink far beyond our capabilities and ambitions – after all of the American governments "best efforts" with unlimited resources they came up with the seven-food group pyramid.

It quickly became apparent that the only hope for being universally successful in our goal to help the average American to surpass the current longevity average of 75 and live to be over 100 was to employ the financially successful and result driven methods used by the veterinary and agricultural industries – preventive herd (population) nutritional supplementation health programs.

No matter who they were, we wanted people to be able to see food and eat it without having to count calories, consider RDA's, become a sociopath and "food combine" (the Diamond's Fit for Life Diets) or to spend their lives shopping for special foods – so we decided to let people eat their traditional religious and cultural diets with impunity, in other words eat what they wanted – what a concept! See food and eat it – Dr. Wallach's See Food Diet was born.

The first task was to focus our culinary effort towards eliminating the negative aspects of human eating habits without tampering with anyone's religious or conceptual choices of dietary needs or goals or their perception of just plain fun foods (i.e.- pizza, tacos, hot dogs, burgers – especially burgers!) Burgers (the 2/3 pound Fuddruckers cooked medium rare) are Dr. Wallach's favorites.

The failure of the hundreds of various "diets" or nutritional programs that have come and gone can be attributed to one common failing - before Dr. Wallach's See food Diet (Chapter 12 - RARE EARTHS: forbidden cures) everyone falsely assumed that "you can get everything you need by eating the basic four food groups" with the admonition to throw in some variety for insurance. The fact is you cannot get everything you need from your four food groups, only the Garden of Eden was perfect and therefore you must supplement completely, properly and consistently if you are to fulfill your genetic potential for leading a slim, healthful and long life.

References

Berger, S.M.: Dr. Berger's Immune Power Diet. NAL Books. New York.1985.

Berry Jr., R.: The Vegetarians. Autumn Press Inc. Brookline, Massachusetts.1979.

Cook, J.: Diet and Your Religion. Woodbridge Press Publishing Co. Santa Barbara, CA. 1976.

D'Adamo, P.J.: Eat Right 4 Your Type. C.P. Putnam's Sons. New York.1996.

Frank, B.S.: No Aging Diet. The Dial Press. New York.1976.

Katahn, M.: The Rotation Diet. W.W. Norton & Co. New York.1986.

McConnell, C. and McConnell, M.: The Mediterranean Diet. W.W. Norton & Co. New York.1987.

Walford, R.: Maximum Lifespan. W.W.Norton & Company. New York. London.1983.

Walford, R.: The 120 Year Diet. Simon & Schuster. New York. 1986.

Wallach, J.D. and Ma, L.: RARE EARTHS: forbidden Cures. Wellness Publications. 1994.

Wallach, J.D. and Ma, L.: Dead Doctors Don't Lie. Wellness Publications. 1999.

Weindruch, R.: Calorie Restriction and Aging. Scientific American. 274:1. 32 –38. Jan. 1996.

Willcox, B.J., Willcox, D. C. and Suzuki, M.: The OKINAWA PROGRAM. Clarkson/Potter. New York. 2001.

Chapter 3

Our Earth is anemic

"It is bad news to learn from our leading authorities that 99% of the American people are deficient in these minerals, and that a marked deficiency in any one of the more important minerals actually results in disease. Any upset of the balance, any considerable lack of one or another element, however microscopic the body requirement might be, and we sicken, suffer, and shorten our lives."

—U.S. Senate Doc. #264
2nd Session, 74th Congress (1936)
Reprinted from Cosmopolitan Magazine

Our Earth is anemic!!! A potentially apocalyptic mixture of chance location of the veins of nutritional minerals, mining, deforestation, agriculture, irrigation and acid rain have shifted, eroded or leached our life-giving and life-sustaining raw materials from our formerly mineral rich land.

It doesn't matter whether one is a creationist or a student of evolution – our immediate mutual problem is that the Earth, our planet, is a limited finite resource for the mineral raw materials that are the basis of all plant, animal and human life as we know it.

Minerals make up as much as two thirds of the total numbers of the essential nutrients necessary to develop properly, reproduce, maintain and repair our physical bodies; therefore, by sheer weight of numbers minerals are important. Secondly, nothing in one's body (biochemical, structural or mechanical) can work without one or more mineral cofactors – nothing! You can't use oxygen, energy, DNA, RNA, chromosomes, protein, carbohydrate, fat, vitamins, minerals, enzymes or hormones without one or more mineral cofactors.

Living organisms procure their mineral and essential element raw materials for reproduction, development, growth and maintenance and for longevity from a thin and fragile blanket of matter and gas on or just above the Earth's crust.

Unfortunately we were given a finite amount of raw materials in the Earth's crust and without the regular impact of large numbers of mineral rich meteors or volcanic eruptions we are forced to conserve and make do with what we have.

There are those who would solve the problem of limited amounts of nutritional minerals in our farm and range soils by re-mineralizing mountain ranges, forests, farms and yes whole continents and oceans to get minerals into our crops and therefore into our human food chain; but put into economic perspective, these dreams are not economically sustainable.

Technically these dreams of redistributing minerals into our farm's soils are possible but are not economically viable. To re-mineralize the Earth's crust for one growing season we would have to annually grind up the equivalent of Mauna Loa, the colossal Hawaiian mountain, and distribute and plow into the soil the resultant rock dust several times each year to coincide with soil preparation and planting. To comprehend the enormity of such a project one has to appreciate that Mauna Loa is the most massive mountain in the world and is also the world's largest volcano.

Mauna Loa rises 13,677 feet above the surface of the Pacific Ocean - an additional 17,000 feet drops from the water's surface to the ocean floor making it technically taller (almost 1 mile taller) than Mt. Everest. Mauna Loa's total mass is 100 times greater than that of Mt. St. Helen in the state of Washington and the lava that forms the massive dome could cover the landmass of the Earth with four feet of mineral dust. As a result of this Herculean effort your hamburger would reach the eye-popping price of $275 per pound and corn would cost $35 per ear - mega sticker shock - it would make $3 a gallon gasoline look pretty cheap!

When Charles Darwin sailed the H.M.S. Beagle to the east

coast of South America in 1833, he recorded the predictable accu-mulation of a fine red dust on his ship each day and correctly deduced that the dust originated from the deserts of west and North Africa. This African dust in its westerly flight, travels all the way to the Amazon and the rainforests where it is essential to replenishing the rain leached mineral poor soils of the rainforests annually.

Man has always realized the enormity of the great and tireless power of the Earth's winds, but their importance to the biological vitality of the Earth and the mineral value of our food is far beyond what we have ever dreamed. There are many wind cur-rents, east to west, that transport great loads of mineral dust across predictable routes, "linking ecosystems hundreds and even thou-sands of miles apart." Billions of tons of mineral-rich dust from the deserts of Asia and Africa annually fertilize oceans, tropical islands and rainforests halfway around the world.

Michael Garstang, professor of meteorology at the University of Virginia in Charlottesville says, "During the violent Amazonian rainstorms, the particulates that originate in African deserts are literally sucked out of the sky." Garstang and his col-leagues calculate that 13,000,000 tons of African and Asian min-eral-rich dust enter the Amazonian soils each season to enrich the rain leached and depleted tropical soils.

The wind-borne African dust adds essential and critical min-erals to help maintain the rainforests productivity. "While the Amazon Basin teems with life, the soil itself lacks reserves of nutrients, especially phosphates, which spur plant growth. The historical record shows that the Amazon rainforest has periodi-cally shrunk to a fraction of its present size, then bounded back again, and the researchers now believe that it expands and con-tracts as the amount of nourishing African dust waxes and wanes with mirror changes in the Saharan desert."

The principle minerals found in the coarse inorganic fraction of soil are directly related to those minerals present in the local parent rock. Minerals that are resistant to weathering (i.e.- quartz) are especially abundant in soils while minerals that weather quickly are rare or are absent. It is therefore possible to calculate the relative age or maturity of a soil covering igneous rocks from its content of primary minerals (i.e.- feldspar, mica, amphiboles and pyroxenes); these relatively soluble minerals are common in young soil and less abundant in mature soils and absent from senescent soils. Soils covering sandstone often contain 90 to 99% quartz; those soils overlying limestone are made up of as much as 80% calcium carbonate.

It is very obvious that minerals are not equally distributed in soils around the earth. The scary part is that fields where our food crops are grown do not contain a uniform blanket of minerals, if they contain any nutritional minerals at all, they occur in veins much like gold and silver or like the chocolate swirls found in chocolate ripple ice cream – at best depending solely on getting the optimal number and amounts of nutritional minerals from food grown in soil is a very risky crap-shoot.

Soils that did have significant amounts of certain nutritional minerals have become depleted as a result of limited thinking. Farmers are paid for tons and bushels, no one gives a farmer any tax break or cash incentive to make sure that we get all of the known 90 essential nutrients.

A comparison of USDA nutrition handbook data published in 1975 with data in 1997 showed a decline in calcium levels in broccoli by 53%. Broccoli also had 38% less vitamin A, 48% less riboflavin, 35% less thiamine and 29% less niacin – similar declines were found for cabbage, carrots, cauliflower, collards, daikon, kale, mustard greens, onions, parsley, turnip greens and watercress.

Crop plants (grains, vegetables, fruits and nuts) take up or "strip-mine" 0.01 kg (10 mg) of minerals per square meter of field per year or approximately 48.4 grams or one tenth of a pound per acre per year – unless the entire plant mass is returned to the soil each year as mulch, the plants will literally "strip-mine" the minerals from the soil to be harvested or carried off and used somewhere else, thus depleting the soil's native reserves of minerals.

Soil conditioners such as animal manure, green manure (cover crops such as clover, beans, etc.), compost, mulch and sphagnum moss increase the soil organic matter level which feeds the soil organisms, increases the percentage of soil atmosphere and the water holding capacity which in turn increases the yields in tons and bushels per acre yet does little or nothing to increase the mineral content of the crops.

Rotating crops or "resting" the field every seventh year as the Bible commands will increase the nitrogen levels of the soil and thus increases the annual yields in tons and bushels but does not appreciably increase the mineral content of the food grown on those fields.

As far as supplements go, vitamins have historically "gotten the glory" and minerals were the stepchildren in the "multi-vitamin" – everyone asks, "Dear, did you take your vitamins today?" Of course they mean, "Dear, did you take your vitamins and minerals today?" As a result of minerals historically being free in nature and can not be manufactured or patented, the medical community rarely looks at minerals as something to prescribe or recommend.

If they do prescribe minerals, doctors want them to be regarded by the patient as prescription drugs such as lithium for depression. Doctors want you to believe that lithium in spring water or a nutritional supplement that heals depression is quackery, but lithium prescribed by them for patients with depression is "good medicine."

Minerals are in fact required by any and all body functions from the basic sub-cellular molecular biological "metallic fingers" of RNA and DNA to electrochemical, catalytic, structural, reproductive, maintenance, repair and a plethora of miscellaneous cellular functions. You can't use **energy** without one or more mineral cofactors; you can't use **oxygen** without one or more mineral cofactors; you can't use **DNA** without one or more mineral cofactors; you can't use **RNA** without one or more mineral cofactors; you can't use **chromosomes** without one or more mineral cofactors; you can't use **enzymes** without one or more mineral cofactors; you can't use **vitamins** without one or more mineral cofactors; you can't use **amino acids, carbohydrates** or **fatty acids** without one or more mineral cofactors; you can't use **anti-oxidants** without one or more mineral cofactors; and you can't use **hormones** (i.e.- estrogen, progesterone, testosterone, adrenal, insulin, thyroid and pituitary) without one or more mineral cofactors!

As important as minerals are to human flesh and the very existence of man, human-kind seems to place more value on machines, software, futures, stocks and bonds, hospitals, doctors, genetically engineered proteins, stem cells, insurance, space travel, military hardware, jet planes, fat free diets and bans on smoking than the human need for the 45 to 60 essential minerals.

The scary part is that we have had official warnings since 1936. Originally published as a Cosmopolitan magazine article by a concerned scientist, U.S. Senate Document #264, was published and entered into the congressional record by the 2nd session of the 74th Congress:

"Do you know that most of us today are suffering from certain dangerous diet deficiencies which cannot be remedied until the depleted soils from which our foods come are brought into proper mineral balance?"

"The alarming fact is that our foods – fruits and vegetables and grains, now being raised on millions of acres of land that no longer contains enough of certain needed minerals, are starving us – no matter how much of them we eat!"

"It is bad news to learn from our leading authorities that 99% of the American people are deficient in these minerals, and that a marked deficiency in any one of the more important minerals actually results in disease. Any upset of the balance, any considerable lack of one or another element, however microscopic the body requirement might be, and we sicken, suffer, and shorten our lives."

In June of 1992 a U.N. Environmental Summit Report (Eco-92) was issued in Rio de Janeiro that documented the decline in numbers of various rare and endangered species, enlarging holes in the ozone layer of our atmosphere, disappearance of tropical rainforests and indigenous peoples – yet the most important and immediate crisis facing the human race was relegated to the few rear pages of the voluminous report – the degradation of our farm and range soils, the decline of the mineral values of our farm and range soils:

Continent	% degraded over 100 years
Africa	74%
Asia	76%
Australia	55%
Europe	72%
North American	85%
South America	76%

In 2001 another warning was put out by saying that soil depletion and degradation continued to occur at an accelerated pace. Additionally the world set out the alarm that the annual bounty of marine fish catch has seriously declined with "over fishing" getting the blame. It is certainly possible theoretically to over fish the oceans, however, with the total human biomass being insignificant compared to the biomass of the oceans which cover 3/5 of the

Earth's surface, a more plausible cause for a decline in the annual catch is that through our zeal to control the great rivers with dams we have cut off the food supply of mineral rich silt to the oceans.

Damming the world's rivers to generate electricity, control flooding and to ensure municipal and agricultural water supplies we have effectively cut off the previously steady supply of silt – the basic food of the oceans. The Hoover Dam blocking the Colorado River in Nevada alone annually catches and accumulates 5 million tons of silt in Lake Mead.

Coral reefs (the oceans "canary in the mine") were the first to feel the effects of a silt deficiency and starvation. Coral reefs are dying at a rapid rate as the microscopic organisms that feed on the silt and are normally consumed by the coral are no longer available – no food, no reef, no small fish, no medium sized fish and no big fish – no fish for human consumption. We have choked off the oceans food supply and starved the ocean into a sterile near death coma.

Animal and fish feed pellets were designed to make up for the deficit of nutritional minerals in soil grown foods – by adding vitamins, minerals, trace minerals, rare earths, amino acids and fatty acids to a uniform dietary pellet every mouthful is guaranteed optimal nutrition. Thus we have complete feed pellets for mice, hamsters, gerbils, guinea pigs, rats, rabbits, dogs, cats, fox, ferrets, pigs, sheep, cattle, horses, poultry, trout, salmon, catfish, talapia, pet birds and primates. Even the most retarded individual representative of any species is guaranteed perfect nutrition if they are fed a commercially prepared diet.

Dr.Wallach's See Food Diet simply incorporates the concept of complete supplementation developed for animals at a cost of $100 billion to ensure optimal nutrition to any and all human diet preferences.

Chapter 4

MINERALS: the currency of life

"Nations endure only as long as their top soil."

—Henry Cantwell Wallace
Professor of Soils
Iowa State College of Agriculture

The classic ancient Old World empires (China, India, Mesopotamia and Egypt) that were the seats of man's transition from ignorant barbarians to modern thinking, governments ruled by law, art and industry shared a basic feature – each was a "hydraulic society." They developed in arid or semiarid plains and valleys fed and more importantly periodically flooded by great rivers that originated in high rocky glacier or snow covered mountains or rainforests.

The hydraulic societies started as isolated bands of hunter-gatherers. In certain locations of high fertility and naturally occurring varieties of high production grains (i.e.- wheat, barley, rye and oats) human populations flourished and grew from small family bands into tribes.

The growing tribes developed and selected the most useful species of wild grains and began to develop agriculture 5,000 years ago. After grain production became predictable and domesticated animals (dogs and pigs) appeared, the most successful tribes became farmers and relegated the value of the bounty of hunting and gathering to dietary supplements.

Large successful tribes developed governments, laws, art, weapons, armies and religions. By means of dams, canals, flood control and drainage projects, governments delivered water and life-giving mineralized silt to their farmer's fields. Applied in steady and unlimited amounts the water borne mineralized silt delivered relatively high yields of highly mineralized food grains per acre – this was possible as long as the primary river flooded annually.

The New World had its early hydraulic-societies too, including the pre-Columbian Mesoamerican cultures of the coasts and highlands of Peru who built complex terrace and aqueduct irrigation systems as well as by the Teotihuacan and the Aztecs' cannibal societies of the Valley of Mexico. These New World hydraulic-societies cultivated maize, potatoes and blue-green alga as carbohydrate sources – their soils lacked the minerals required to raise livestock and maintain human health so they developed complex ritualistic cannibal societies to justify the wholesale consumption of human flesh and bones as their main protein and mineral source.

The settling of the Americas by Europeans introduced dry land farming that relied on seasonal rain and snow as water sources for agriculture – land was free for the taking, all one had to do was clear the forests or plow the prairies. Unfortunately, without the annual flooding and supply of mineralized silt supplied in the great flood plains of the hydraulic societies and smaller river bottoms (bottom land) the land of the great plains "played out" in five to 10 years forcing the small farm family or "sod buster" to pack up and move west to new and still "virgin" or untilled prairie.

The first signs that the soil was "played out" did not appear as obvious changes in the crops, but rather in the humans and livestock relying on the land as a food source. The newborn infants, calves, lambs and pigs were underweight, weak and died; women, cows, ewes and sows became infertile; they developed pneumonia, consumption (tuberculosis), scarlet fever, diphtheria and flu killing people and animals of all ages during the winter; adult humans and animals died of new unheard of diseases many years before their expected time for death. To escape these terrible places of death and despair, people unceremoniously packed up and moved west.

Those sodbusters that could not or would not leave their exhausted homesteads, finally observed declines in production followed by outright crop failure, erosion and dust bowl formation. This scenario occurred over and over on small individual farms of America finally culminating in a total ecological collapse that produced the great dust bowls of Oklahoma, Texas, Nebraska, Iowa and Kansas in the 1930's.

The recurrent problem of the soil "playing out" was not a mystery but an accepted part of the process of life and death in dry land farming plains communities. There were numerous ways in which to slow the process including the biblical method of letting the land rest every seventh year, the application of animal and green manure (cover crops and plant waste) to replace used up organic matter, cover crops to reduce wind erosion, hold in moisture and add growth stimulating nitrogen to the fields; composting plant and animal wastes to add to the humus content of the soil; the application of guano (large quantities of nitrogen-rich droppings of shore birds) and lastly the advent of commercial NPK fertilizers. These procedures and applications only slowed or delayed the process of crop nutritional failure while keeping tonnage and bushel production up.

While nearly all farmers understand the necessity to maintain the optimal level of organic material and humus in their fields to sustain tonnage production, very few realize the slow insidious leaching and depletion or mining of the life giving minerals from their land – after all we pay them for tons and bushels not for an analysis of minimal levels of various minerals in each carrot, potato, broccoli or bushel of wheat. This belief is summed up in a statement by a professor of soils from Iowa State College of

Agriculture Henry Cantwell Wallace (George Washington Carver's favorite teacher and editor of the Wallace's Farmer), "Nations endure only as long as their topsoil." The statement should relay the message that "Nations endure only as long as nutritional minerals are available in their topsoil."

It is projected that by the year 2050 there will be somewhere between 800,000 and 5 million Americans over the age of 100 and by 2100 there will be more than 12 billion humans on Earth – there is no way that our farm soils can sustain the mineral nutritional value of our soils, our food or ourselves. Genetic engineering, better varieties of wheat, rice and corn and perhaps even better fertilizer will produce more tons and bushels of crops that are tastier, contain more vitamins ("Golden rice") and have longer shelf life ("Frankenfoods") – but they will not sustain us, they will not prevent birth defects caused by mineral deficiencies, they will not totally nurture our babies, maintain and heal our adult bodies, support our 100 year olds and they will not forestall learning deficits, antisocial, psychotic or criminal behavior.

A review of mineral deficiency diseases would be a book in of itself so we will ask the reader to go to *RARE EARTHS: forbidden cures* to appreciate the magnitude of devastation that mineral deficiencies wreak on America's unsuspecting population. You can't get everything you need from your basic four food groups!

The animal industry has long been able to solve, prevent and eliminate health problems in animals with complete prepared diets, prevent and eliminate infertility and birth defects by means of special supplement programs and special prepared diets for animals with heart disease, diabetes, gastrointestinal disease, kidney disease, liver disease, arthritis, osteoporosis, cancer, Alzheimer's disease, fibromyalgia, etc.

Since 1978, Wallach has been using preformulated supplement programs in humans designed for treating specific diseases – animal supplement and premixed special foods used for human disease. In September of 2001 food manufacturers have now "discovered" and project that they will in the near future use specialized prepared diets for human diseases based on genetics – enter nutrigenomics! Unfortunately, few if any of the diseases thought to be genetic by the medical profession are genetic – again, close, but no cigar!

Chapter 5

Age Beaters

"The first cup of tea moistens my lips and throat, the second cup breaks my loneliness, the third cup searches my barren mind but to find volumes of wandering thoughts. The fourth cup raises a slight perspiration – All the wrongs of life pass away through my pores. At the fifth cup I am purified. The sixth cup, and I can hear the immortals call. The seventh cup – ah, but I could take no more – let me ride on this sweet breeze to the land of the immortals."

—Lotung, a poet
T'ang dynasty

All species have a genetic potential or upper limit for longevity – mice 700 days, dogs 23 years, horses 32 years, elephant 45 years, chimpanzee 52 years and man more than 200 years – whether or not an individual of that species reaches or fulfills their genetic potential for longevity depends on two basic concepts.

1) Avoiding the "land mines" or eliminating unnecessary and wasteful death from predators, muggers, terrorists, road accidents, smoking, alcohol consumption to excess, avoiding the use of illegal and prescription drugs, avoid carbonated drinks and caffeine, avoid fried foods, cooking oils and margarines, do not cook your meat well done, reduce or better yet eliminate sugar and carbohydrates, avoiding chemicals and toxic wastes in our food, air and water and lastly avoid going to a doctor for problems that you can safely handle yourself!

2) Do those positive things necessary to make it beyond 120 including the daily supplementation of each of the 90 known essential nutrients (60 minerals, 16 vitamins, 12 essential amino acids and 3 essential fatty acids) in optimal amounts, consume isolated and natural sources of antioxidants daily, drink eight to 10 glasses of pure water each day, eat high quality animal protein including eggs, red meat, poultry, fish and whey and use herbs and herbal medicines when possible instead of over the counter and prescription drugs.

Assuming that you successfully negotiate around and avoid the "landmines" of life, then health and longevity depend upon how faithfully one takes in the optimal amounts of the 90 essential nutrients necessary for health and longevity each and every day – longevity is not a guaranteed genetic destiny or an unwitting lottery but a prize that can be consciously achieved or won by anyone who is committed to living to be 120.

An analogy to our genetic potential for longevity is the engine of a Mercedes which is a wonder of German automotive engineering – the engine is designed to run 300,000 miles before it needs a major overhaul or needs to be replaced, yet if you the owner/driver don't maintain the Mercedes engine by supplying the essential coolants, lubricants and motor oil that wonderful engine designed to run 300,000 miles won't run 50 miles. Without oil or coolant even a Mercedes won't make it to its engineered potential (genetic potential) of 300,000 miles (200 human years).

Dr. Alexis Carrel (1912), a Nobel Prize recipient, grew fibroblasts (stem cells) from chicken hearts in flasks. He fed the fibroblasts with extracts of blended and filtered chicken embryo and the heart fibroblasts (stem cells) kept multiplying and growing for 34 years (2 years after Carrel's own death).

Carrel's colleagues got bored with the experiment and threw the stem cells out, but not before he developed the theory that stem cells are inherently immortal if fed a perfect diet and kept in a perfect environment.

Unfortunately Dr. Leonard Hayflick came along and used an incomplete artificial growth media with major mineral deficiencies for propagating human stem cells – in his experiment (faulted from the start) human stem cells could only divide 50 times before dying out and showing accumulations of ceroid lipofuscin (oxidized lipid pigments of aging that indicate a vitamin E, selenium and antioxidant deficiencies). Hayflick attributed Carrel's stem cell "immortality" to contamination of the nutritional media by embryonic stem cells from the chick embryo, rather than admitting that the nutritionally deficient diet media prematurely ended the life of his stem cells. The 50-replication limit is known in academic circles as the "Hayflick limit."

The association between maximizing one's longevity and the intake of optimal amounts of essential nutrients is well documented in the laboratory for many species of animals. Humans in several isolated Third World cultures in far-flung corners of the earth have well documented good health and exceptional longevity without access to western medicine. While the people of the long-lived cultures do not each have a PhD in biochemistry or nutrition they have by serendipity set up their homelands in an idyllic biochemical Garden of Eden. These Third World countries are superficially quite different, however, it is their similarities or common denominators that give them their healthful longevity.

There are well-known human cultures whose peoples routinely live to their healthful maximum genetic potential for longevity – the fact that all the long-lived cultures are third world countries is significant (the longest average longevity recorded for an industrialized nation is 81.2 held by the Okinawa Japanese). The Tibetans in the northwest of China, the Hunzakut of eastern Pakistan, the Russian Georgians (and their sister cultures of Armania, Azerbaijan and Abkhazia in the Caucasus Mountains) and certain regions of Turkey, the Vilcabamba in the Andes of Ecuador, the Titicaca of the Peruvian Andes and the Okinawa Japanese are world famous for their high average lifespan and large percentages of centenarians.

The common denominators of the long-lived cultures include:

1) Food choices are simple; none of the long-lived cultures are vegetarians (they eat an average of 10 to 15 pounds of animal products (milk, cheese, butter, eggs, fish, poultry, red meat) per month; total daily caloric intakes range from 1,200 to 1,800 per day, they consume large amounts of antioxidants (catechins) in the form of green and black tea.

2) There is no heavy industry to pollute the air, water or food.

3) Only natural fertilizer (manure, human feces, plant debris and highly mineralized Glacial Milk or kelp) is employed.

4) Western allopathic medicine was not historically available to these cultures and thus they avoided major land mines.

The Tibetans:

The Tibetans were the inspiration for the Pulitzer Prize winning book by James Hilton, *The Lost Horizon*. Tibet's old people are found on Chang Tang or the northern plateau, elevation 15,000 feet, which consists of salt lakes fed by glaciers from the eastern slopes of the Himalayan Mountains. This mountain culture has about 500,000 people who are devout Buddhists. The Tibetans are a mix of nomadic herdsmen, salt merchants, farmers and great cavalrymen on camel or horse.

Tibet makes up nearly 10% of China's land mass and was founded in the 7th century by King Songtsan Gambo. The Chinese government took over Tibet in 1950 by sending a large army to establish a military governor. Since 1965 the region has been administered by China and known as the Tibetan Autonomous Region (T.A.R.) of China.

The Tibetan herdsman build their corrals, huts and roads out of salt bricks carefully cut from dried salt lakes on the top of the plateau; they hunt Marco Polo Sheep, antelope, gazelle, wild asses and yak.

The yak, which translates to "wealth" provides meat, sausage, milk, cheese, yogurt, butter, wool, skins and animal power for plowing, riding or for carrying freight.

The staple Tibetan diet consists of "tsampa," a smelly hand-mixed paste of lightly toasted barley flour, yak butter, salt and black tea. Tsampa is supplemented with turnips, cabbage, potatoes, trout, egg omelettes and beans.

Tibetans routinely drink 30 to 40 medium sized cups of black or green tea daily (a great source of catechins or ECGC antioxidants that are 100 times more potent in neutralizing free radicals than vitamin C) because the high elevation is extremely dry requiring a high fluid intake. Each cup of tea is flavored with a chunk of rock salt the size of a concord grape and two pats of yak or goat butter.

The Tibetan capital city of Lhasa (translates to "Place of the Gods") was the inspiration for James Hilton's legendary city of Shangri-La. The city is found at an elevation of 12,000 feet; daily temperatures can fluctuate as much as 80 to 100 degrees.

In the center of old Lhasa is the Jokhang, the holiest shrine in Tibet. The Jokhang, built in 650 A.D. is the "Mecca" to the Tibetan Buddhists – many of the faithful would trek through the mountains for years to come and pray at this holy site.

In the mountains west of Lhasa is Drepung, a gigantic monastery that houses 10,000 monks, 25,000 surfs and assistants working 185 estates and tending more than 200 pastures.

The Potala, "High Heavenly Realm," is a sprawling mountain top palace of the Dalai Lama (translates to "Ocean of Wisdom" and represents the living prophet of the Buddhist faith and the inspiration for the ancient prophet in James Hilton's The Lost Horizon) built into the mountain 700 feet above Lhasa. The Potala is famous for its 1,000 rooms, 10,000 altars, 200,000 statues of Budda and the eight gold gilded tombs of past Dalai Lamas.

South of Lhasa are tens of thousands of acres of terraces fed and watered by mineral-rich "Glacial milk" which originates in the Himalayan glaciers and supplies an endless source of minerals.

Li-Ching-Yun is said to have lived to the age of 256 years and he outlived 23 wives! Li of Kaihsien, in the province of Szechwan, China was born in 1677 and died in 1933 at the age of 256 years (and was the inspiration for the 200 year-old leader of Hilton's Shangri-La).

Professor Wu-Chung-Chien, the dean of the Department of Education, of the Minkuo University claims to have found records showing that Li was in fact born in 1677 (the Chinese have the most complete and accurate of all census records in the history of man), and that on his 150th birthday (1827), he was congratulated by the Chinese Imperial government. Fifty years later, in 1877, Li was sent another official congratulations on his 200th birthday. Fifty years later, at the age of 250 years, Li lectured to a thousand medical students in Beijing on the art of living a long healthy life. Li's advice for living a long healthful life included "Keep a quiet heart, sit like a tortoise, sleep like a dog." Li sold herbs during his first 100 years of life.

London Times May 8, 1933

Telegrams in Brief – A telegram from Chungking in the province of Szechwan, China states that Li-Ching-Yun, reputed to be the oldest man in China and presumably the world, has died at Kiah-Sien, at the alleged age of 256. – Reuters.

New York Times May 6, 1933

Li-Ching-Yun – Dead
Gave his age as 197

The Russian Georgians:

The Russian Georgians as well as the Abkazians, Azerbaijanis and Armanians are found at the timberline of the Caucasus

Mountains, which have peaks of 12,434 to 13,274 feet above sea level. They live in simple stone houses without electricity, their blood pressure is typically 104/72 at age 100; women continue to have children after age 52; they typically drink an eight ounce glass of vodka with breakfast and have a large glass of wine with lunch and dinner. Almost all of the "old people" are from rural backgrounds or occupations such as farmers, shepherds and/or hunters.

The culturally divergent centenarians, from the Caucasus Mountains, are dispersed between the coasts of the Black Sea and the Caspian Sea and additionally in mountain villages at or above 4,500 feet above sea level. This region supports over 500,000 people of whom 4,500 to 5,000 are over the age of 100 years.

1,844 centenarians in Russian Georgia ....(39/100,000)
2,500 centenarians in Azerbaijan.................(84/100,000)
Vilcabamba...(1/100)
United States (1900) ....(1/100,000)
              (1950) ....(3/100,000)
              (2001) ....(10/100,000)
Okinawa...(34/100,000)

Mejid Agayev celebrated his 140th birthday February 12, 1975. Agayev was the oldest living citizen in the Azerbaijani village of Tikyaband that bragged of having 54 people over the age of 100 years!

According to a National Geographic gerantologist (January 1973) the oldest known living person was from the Caucasus region of the U.S.S.R. He was Shirali Mislimov; at age 167 he still worked in the village tea plantation in the small village of Barzavu on the Iranian border. Mislimov turned 168 in May of 1973 and reportedly died just a few days before his 169th birthday.

The Azerbaijanis feel that youth is up to 80 years of age, 80 to 100 years is middle age and at 100 to 160 years they are seniors. Many married couples are married for more than 100 years.

A study of over 15,000 Azerbaijanis over the age of 100 showed only married individuals attained advanced age and still have an active sex life.

Work relegated to centenarians included weeding fields, feeding livestock, shepherds, picking tea, washing laundry, housework and babysitting.

Women over 100 years of age usually had between four and 15 children during their child bearing years.

The staple diet of the Caucasus region includes chicken, mutton, beef, goat milk, cheese, yogurt, butter, bread, tomatoes, cucumbers, green onions, garlic, fruit, pita bread, boiled corn meal mush (abusta), red pepper, tea, wine and salt. Their total caloric intake per day ranges between 1,800 and 1,900. Their terraced fields have been irrigated with highly mineralized glacial milk for over 2,500 years.

The Vilcabambas:

Ecuador's star-shaped "Sacred Valley of Longevity" (Vilcabamba) is actually five valleys that converge and sit between two Andean Mountains at 12,434 feet above sea level. The western skyline of Vilcabamba is dominated by the summit of Mandango, the tallest mountain whose glaciers supply the mineral rich "glacial milk" which is used to irrigate the terraced fields. The "glacial milk" originating from the high peaks of the Podocarpus National Park pours into the Rio Yambala, which converges with the Chamba River, which is also used for irrigation.

In 1971 an official census revealed nine people over the age of 100 years in the population of 819 or an astounding one centenarian per 100 people! Miguel Carpio at age 123 was the oldest living Vilcabamban found at the census – he still smoked, drank wine and "chased women."

The staple diet of the Vilcabamba Indian includes corn, beans, goat meat, pork, chicken, eggs, milk, cheese and a soup known as repe, which is made from bananas, beans, white cheese, salt and lard. The average total calorie intake for the Vilcabamba is 1,200 to 1,800 calories per day.

The Titicaca:

Legend says that the first Incas came to earth on an island in Lake Titicaca to start what was to become the most advanced civilization of pre-Columbian America.

Titicaca is found in the Andean highlands of Peru at 12,506 feet above sea level. The main city of Titicaca is Puno (population 32,000); the people of the Altiplano (high plains) are divided into the pure Indians and the "mestizos" who are a mix of Indian and Spanish. The treeless hills that form the "Altiplano" surrounding Lake Titicaca are covered with "pata pata," or stone terraces built by the Incas to provide level farming areas and as catchments for the mineral rich "Glacial milk" roaring from the great Andean mountain, Mt. Cardillera Real with which they irrigated their crops.

The Okinawans:

Okinawa is an archipelago made up of 161 islands that are strung over 800 miles of the Pacific Ocean between the Japanese main island and Taiwan and is known as the "Galapagos of the East." The original Okinawa kingdom was an independent state – it only became a Japanese annex in 1879.

Okinawans currently enjoy the longest average lifespan of any Japanese subculture. The Okinawan's average lifespan only began to lengthen to the current high level after World War II. Okinawan women average 86 years of age at death, men 78 years for an Okinawan average longevity of 81.2 - the oldest documented average lifespan of any known culture. The Okinawans currently boast 34 centenarians per 100,000 people.

In the fishing and farming village of Ogimi six of its 3,500 residents are 100 years of age or older – that's a whopping 171 centenarians per 100,000 people in the village. A stone marker on the outskirts of Ogimi facing the sea displays a carved Okinawan quotation that says, "At 70 you are still a child, at 80 a young man or woman. And if at 90 someone from heaven invites you over, tell him: 'just go away, and come back when I am 100.'"

Cardiovascular disease is rare (82% lower than U.S. rate); breast cancer is so infrequent (82% lower than U.S. rate) that mammograms are not commonly done; prostate cancer is unheard of (86% lower than U.S. rate) and the three top killers of western populations are recorded in Okinawans at the lowest rate of any culture in the world!

According to western doctors the Japanese do everything wrong – 68% smoke heavily; they fry everything (rice, tempura, vegetables); they eat raw fish with worms in it (sushi); the Okinawan elders consume seven grams of salt per day, the main island Japanese consume 12 grams of salt per day; and the United States dropped two atomic bombs on them – the Japanese have absorbed more radiation per person than any other culture (the U.S. dropped two atomic bombs on them to end WWII), yet they live 4.1 years longer than Americans and have half the cancer rate.

The traditional Okinawan diet contains less than 2,000 calories and is considerably different from the USDA's seven-food group pyramid. The Okinawans cook their food at low heat and very slowly, stir frying on low heat compared to the Japanese who tend to deep-fry a lot of their dishes with high heat. Okinawan elders eat seven servings of vegetables each day, seven servings of grain per day, two servings of soy per day, three servings of Omega- 3 rich fish per week, two percent of their daily diet is seaweed and kelp and modest amounts of meat and eggs each day.

The Okinawans eat significant amounts of seaweed each day (notably three times the Japanese average), which supplies a large quantity and variety of minerals including calcium, magnesium, iron, zinc, copper, iodine, tin and arsenic. Mineral rich kelp is reported by the Okinawans to re-color gray hair, re-grow hair, lower elevated blood pressure to normal levels and successfully treat arthritis.

There are more than 2,500 species of marine seaweed which includes **kombu**, a brown kelp gathered primarily from the cool waters of the northern Japanese island of Hokkaido; **nori** is a red seaweed, that turns black when it is dried – it is used to wrap sushi, wrap rice balls, eaten as dried strips for breakfast (the Irish and Welsh call it laver and use it to make flat cakes); **hijiki** is a black seaweed that is eaten simmered with mixed vegetables; **wakame** is a kelp that tastes like spinach lasagna and is used in soup, salads and a wakame/buckwheat noodle known as wakame soba. Seaweed and tofu "mooi tofu" mixes are a particular favorite tofu dish of the Ogimi villagers.

The Japanese and Okinawans claim that their secret weapon against aging is green tea. Green tea was described as the "The Cure-All of Cure-Alls" in the September 1998 issue of Investor's Business Daily. They reported on a study by the Case Western Reserve University Medical School (Cleveland, Ohio) that compared the cancer rate of two groups of laboratory mice fed chemicals that cause cancer. One group received green tea the other did not. At the end of the study the green tea group developed 90% less cancer.

The substances or phytochemicals in green tea credited with the anti-cancer properties are called catechins or EGCGs – they are potent antioxidants that are 100 times more potent than vitamin C and 25 times more potent in neutralizing free- radicals than vitamin E.

The newer generations of Okinawans have become "westernized" in their lifestyle and dietary habits and therefore unfortunately do not share in the longevity benefits exhibited by the "old ones." Okinawans that migrate to other countries and take on their new homelands habits and diets do not show the historical Okinawan health and longevity. Over 100,000 Okinawans moved to Brazil and adopted the eating habits of their new homeland – their average age dropped from the Okinawan average of 81.2 to 64. It is quite obvious that the longevity and health benefits shown by the "old ones" is not a genetically based benefit but dependent only on dietary habits and local food sources.

Chapter 6

The American Centenarians

"American centenarians are fiesty, drink lots of whole milk, do not pay attention to cholesterol, often smoke and have no history of exercise."

—Leonard W. Poon
Georgia Centenarian Study

In 1900 there was one American centenarian per 100,000 of population, today there are 10 per 100,000. There were 2,300 American 100 year olds in 1950, 78,000 American centenarians in 2001, 1,535 in the state of Michigan and 3,573 in the state of Florida (145 of which are over the age of 110) – there is no doubt that more and more Americans are going to live to be 100, in fact many will live to be more than 150 years of age and they are already alive today. Demographers project there will be some-where between 800,000 and 5 million centenarians in the United States by 2050.

Ralph Charles still flies his Aronca Defender single engine plane solo at the age of 100 years with no restrictions on his pilots license or health papers; Harold Stilson from Deerfield Beach, Florida hit his 6th hole in one (a 108 yard par 3 hole) at the age of 101 years; Harley Potter still plays golf weekly at the age of 103 and he only learned how to play golf at age 92; Jeanne Calment of France wrote and recorded a best selling CD of 100 year old French folk music at age 121 years; Shirali Mislimov of

Azerbaijan still worked as a field hand harvesting tea at the age of 168.

Many say they would not want to live to be a 100 years of age because of fears of being disabled and winding up in a nursing home hooked up to wires, tubes and monitors – forget those fears, because up to 75 percent of 100 year olds are fit both mentally and physically because the sick and infirm died when they were in their 50s, 60's and 70s!

Remember, its not medical science that's going to get you to 100 years of age, its what you eat, what foods and lifestyles you avoid and how completely and how faithfully you supplement with the 90 essential nutrients.

A Harvard study published in December of 1997 revealed that the percentage of Americans over the age of 65 and centenarians were not equally distributed across America. The county by county Harvard search showed that the upper Midwestern part of the United States produces the greatest percentage of older people over the age of 65 and the greatest percentage of centenarians; the southeastern part of the United States and the eastern seaboard has the shortest life spans of Americans and has the highest rates of cancer, stroke and heart attacks – as a result the eastern seaboard is known as "the cancer, stroke and heart attack belt of America."

In 1895 Americans averaged 48 years of age, which increased to 75.5 in 1975. While medical doctors would like to claim credit for the 30-year increase in the average life span for Americans it is clear that nothing that doctors have done has added ten seconds to the American life span.

There has not be a single heart transplant recipient live to be a 100 years of age and 85 percent of heart transplant recipients die before their new hearts first anniversary. Antibiotics save kids from strep – throat, scarlet fever and diphtheria and old men from bouts of pneumonia but don't add 50 years to the average American's live span.

The increase in American life span from 48 to 75.5 is the

direct result of individual, city, county, state and federal public health advances – clean water, sewers, food inspection and personal hygiene – these engineering feats and personal hygiene practices are the real heroes of our current state of health and longevity (average age of 75.5).

Clean food and water, sewers and personal hygiene carried us only so far in our quest for health and longevity – 75.5. After marking time at 75.5 (give or take a few years) since 1950, it is glaringly obvious that there is yet another piece missing, the piece necessary to catapult the average American longevity to the next level – an average American life span of 100 years!

In April of 1990 the World Health Organization and the Center for Disease Control ranked Americans 17th in longevity amongst the top 32 industrialized nations in the world – 16 other countries had citizens that lived longer than we did! The study was rerun ten years later and reported in June of 2000 that Americans had dropped to a world ranking of 24th for longevity – there were then 23 other countries whose peoples lived longer than we did in the year 2000. Why, are we going backwards when it comes to longevity instead of gaining on the countries that have less food, lower quality food, less money and less medical technology than we do?

It is important to remember that in 1998 the entire world spent $2.7 trillion for health care and of that total the United States spent $1.5 trillion – more than half. In June of 2000 the WHO ranked the top 50 countries in the world for the quality of health care - the American health care system ranked 37th for quality. We do in fact have the most expensive and the most technologically advanced health care system in the world but it is far from being the best! In a results orientated comparison our American health care system stinks – we don't even show up on the radar screen!

The obvious question is who was number one and what did their people and governments do different from us and how do we get there from here. The Japanese were number one in average longevity both in 1990 (79.1) and in 2000 (74.9).

It is of special interest to note that according to western doctors the Japanese do everything wrong when it comes to a healthy lifestyle. The average Japanese smokes more than almost any other people or country on earth; they fry everything (rice, tempura, stir fry, etc.); they eat raw fish with parasites in it (sushi); they consume 12 grams of salt each day; they treat themselves with traditional oriental remedies for most diseases (acupuncture, massage, meditation, herbs, vitamins and minerals) and we dropped two atomic bombs on them – they have been exposed to more radiation per person than any other culture on earth, yet they live an average of four years longer than Americans do and have a significantly lower cancer rate (50% - 80% less) and half the heart disease than Americans.

Highlights from the 2000 U.S. census show that centenarians have increased from 1990 by 35%, they also indicate that California, America's most populated state had 5,341 centenarians or 0.016% of its population. The state with the highest percentage of centenarians is South Dakota at 0.033% of their population centenarians. Although American women continue to outnumber American men in percentage of individuals over age 65, men have made gains from 67 men per 100 women in 1990 to 70 men per 100 women in 2000.

The Mormons have historically lived longer than the average American by as much as 10 years living on the average to 85 years of age; they have a significantly lower cancer and cardiovascular disease rate. These health and longevity benefits enjoyed by the Mormons are attributed to their simple health rules – avoid smoking, alcohol and caffeine!

The next generation of Mormons may not continue to enjoy their longevity advantage as caffeine is found in soft drinks, chocolate, sports drinks, energy bars and energy drinks.

The Seventh Day Adventist have health laws similar to those of the Mormons and in addition to the restrictions the Mormons use, they also exclude pork – as a result they live to about 85 just like the Mormons.

The shortest-lived Americans are black Americans, low income white Americans and Hispanics – they do not avoid alcohol, smoking, pork, fried food, margarine, processed meats, burnt animal fat or caffeine, they tend to eat diets high in fried food and high in carbohydrates. Black, poor white and Hispanic cultures do not traditionally supplement with vitamins and minerals. As a result of their poor eating habits and lack of a consistent nutrient supplement program, the Hispanic, poor whites and black Americans have higher rates of arthritis, osteoporosis, cancer, hypertension, heart disease and diabetes than whites and Asians – the difference is not genetic, its how and what we eat.

To level the playing field of longevity in America all of us, every race, every culture needs to supplement with all 90 essential nutrients. One University of Iowa study on 400 Iowans 79 and older living independently in rural areas revealed that 80% of those who responded consumed inadequate amounts of four or more nutrients. Seventy-five percent of those people consumed too little folate; 83% did not get enough vitamin D and 63% got too little calcium. Other nutrients commonly in short supply were vitamin E, magnesium, vitamin B6, vitamin C and zinc.

In another report on better nutrition among the elderly published by Memorial University of Newfoundland showed that a nutrient supplement with modest amounts of 18 vitamins, minerals and trace minerals could improve the cognitive function of people older than 65. Investigators were struck by the cost-effectiveness and simplicity of a nutritional supplement's ability to prevent or delay illness and functional decline in the elderly. Based on their findings, investigators calculated that for every dollar spent on nutrient supplements, $28 would be saved in health-care costs!

If we could make complete supplementation programs universal in America we could eliminate arthritis, osteoporosis, hypertension and adult onset type II diabetes within 90 days and significantly reduce the cancer rate (reduce by 65% - 462%) within five years – unfortunately this scenario is not in the financial interest of the medical profession or the pharmaceutical industry so we can expect little or no cooperation, encouragement or help from them for a dramatic change in the direction of health care philosophy.

The universal use of serious supplement programs necessary to eliminate the major disease killers in America will have to be a grass roots program of the people, there will be no help from government agencies, public health services, insurance, doctors or private medical services.

Pharmaceutical companies pay out $14 billion each year in advertising, incentives, perks and outright kickbacks to doctors to encourage them to use drugs to treat disease – no one pays doctors a single penny to use nutrition and herbs, therefore they don't! We all would like to think our doctors are altruistic and their primary goal is to heal and cure us and that their great life styles and high incomes are just an unsolicited benefit of doing good work, however, one has to remember that there are no laws requiring doctors to cure you even if a cure is available, so they don't.

Middle age and older individuals are often willing to spend great sums of money and put out great levels of effort just to look good. They will get plastic surgery to make their nose smaller or their breasts larger or BOTOX injections to reduce the size of wrinkles in hopes of enhancing their life, however, they quickly learn that the vanity of just looking good doesn't cut it.

This reality is that looking good alone is not the answer to having a great life after the age of fifty and living healthfully to 100 years, yet the willingness of humans to pay everything just to look good is best illustrated by the classic Oscar Wilde (1891) poem - The Picture of Dorian Gray:

> "How sad it is!" murmured Dorian Gray with his eyes still fixed upon his own portrait. "How sad it is! I shall grow old, and horrible, and dreadful. But this picture will remain always

young. It will never be older than this particular day of June....If it were only the other way! If it were I who was to be always young, and the picture that was to grow old! For that – for that – I would give everything! Yes, there is nothing in the whole world I would not give! I would give my soul for that!"

Good health is an absolutely essential factor for a happy and healthy sex life after the age of 60 years. Depression, pain, serious disease, physical debility and general weakness are common causes of a failed sex life in seniors. The vigor, strength and stamina necessary for a healthy sex life can be obtained and maintained well beyond 100 years of age by an intense nutritional supplement program not with plastic surgery and not with cosmetics.

A common American myth surrounding the life style of seniors is that older people don't have sex or don't have good sex. This myth is just that, a myth! Right now as the baby boomers are reaching their late fifties, there is a senior sexual revolution going on in America. About 10 million men are on Viagra prescriptions for erection enhancement and it is obvious that seniors are not asexual. Viagra is providing a sexual revolution for middle age and older men similar to the sexual revolution that was provided for women by birth control pills. There are herbal alternatives to Viagra including pygeum, saw palmetto, pumpkin seed and gingko and with the herbs there is no risk of death!

From age 65 to 80, approximately one out of four men have trouble getting and maintaining erections; after the age of 80 years, one out of two have erection problems. Viagra can work effectively for 66% of the men suffering from erection problems.

Older men can make excellent lovers because as they age they can control and delay ejaculation which gives women a greater chance of having an orgasm.

Women who were able to have orgasms as younger women continue to have orgasms after the age of 80 years. Women who are willing to stop having sex after the age of 80 were often ones who didn't enjoy sex when they were younger.

Lastly, American centenarians must take control of the imple-
mentation of their own health care direction and control; they
must look at doctors as technicians necessary only to perform certain procedures and services that one can't do for them selves
(i.e.- surgery, prescriptions, etc.). If it is in fact necessary to see a
physician, then the senior patient must maintain certain rights to
prevent abuse by the unscrupulous doctor:

- Cures must be used when cures are known to be available.
- Preventative procedures must be used when prevention is
  available.
- Seniors have the right to choose the doctor of their choice.
- Doctors must give full disclosure of all options available –
  even those considered to be alternative.
- Seniors must get second opinions from doctors not financially associated with the first doctor.
- Seniors must have access to the scorecard of each doctor's
  successes and failures on an annual basis (i.e.- killed,
  injured, infected, etc.).
- Seniors must be fully informed of a doctor's relationship to
  insurance companies, pharmaceutical companies and the
  annual dollar amount of kickbacks and perks they receive.
- Seniors should have an instant 24-hour appeal process if
  insurance claims are denied.

Chapter 7

Wallach's Law: Weight Loss and Weight Management

"Ninety-five percent of all Americans of all age groups are minerally deficient."

—U.S. Department of Agriculture

Obesity and weight problems are synonymous with Americans. Nibble, nibble, nibble all the way home. "Pica" is a seeking, a craving with licking and chewing behavior that has its genesis in mineral deficiencies – interestingly enough neither vitamin deficiency, protein deficiency or calorie deficiency initiates this "pica" behavior, nor will supplementing vitamins or eating sugar, carbohydrate, fat or protein quench it! Only the consumption of the essential minerals in optimal amounts can prevent and eliminate cravings, pica, cribbing and the munchies! Eliminate cravings and you automatically and easily eliminate excess weight!

It is not genetic, it is not your glands, it is not lack of self control, it is these mineral deficiencies that are the basic root cause of obesity, deal with the mineral deficiencies and weight loss occurs without effort and keeping the weight off is assured.

Weight loss products and meal substitutes that contain sugar, caffeine and fiber only intensify the cravings and binging on the weight problem by reducing absorption and increasing the rate of loss of minerals. The law, "Wallach's Law" of weight loss and weight management, is simple – take in 60 minerals and you will lose weight; lose minerals and you will gain weight. Wallach's Law is as predictable as gravity!

Since American soils are critically deficient and depleted in minerals it is no surprise that pica, cribbing, munchies and cravings dominate the American scene. Americans are universally minerally deficient – dieters, athletes, vegetarians, meat eaters, embryos, toddlers, children, teenagers, young adults, middle aged and seniors are starved for minerals.

According to the U.S.D.A. 95% of all Americans of all age groups are minerally deficient. That means that 95% of all newborns, toddlers, preteens, teens, young adults, middle age and seniors are minerally deficient. No wonder 60% of Americans are overweight and 30% are obese.

"Cribbing" in animals signals the farmer, rancher and husbandry man that their farm animals are minerally deficient – they chew on fences, the feed box, the barn door and eat dirt. Farmers give their livestock minerals to save their life, keep the veterinary bills down and the keep them from literally eating the barn!

The "munchies" or the "you just can't eat one" behavior in humans is the same as cribbing in animals. The munchies urge in people has the same genesis as the cribbing urge in animals – the same behavior by another name still has the same root cause – mineral deficiencies!

The snack food and fast food industries are aware of this relationship between the munchies, pica, cribbing, cravings, sugar and carbohydrate binges and salt hunger and they use it to their advantage by liberally salting or sweetening or adding phosphates to their products – "you just can't eat one."

Unfortunately for us our bodies temporarily translates sugar, salt and phosphate consumption as a fulfillment of the craving for nutritional minerals (i.e.- if we lack iron, ice, salt or sugar will temporarily satisfy our pica behavior initiated by the iron deficiency).

Historically, the consumption of salt to satisfy a pica behavior was of value because salt was not processed and bleached and did often times contain trace minerals and Rare Earths. Today, salt consumption, although contrary to popular medical belief, is not in and of itself harmful; it does present the problem of allowing our bodies to think we are getting minerals (the mineral equivalent of the "empty calorie diets"- i.e.- processed food calories without vitamins).

Farmers and husbandry men use the salt hunger of animals to ensure the consumption of trace minerals by incorporating trace minerals in salt blocks containing 85% sodium chloride. A salt content of anything less than 85% sodium chloride in a trace mineral salt block will be ignored - even if they have major mineral deficiencies.

"Cribbing" is the name given to a particular form of pica behavior in domestic animals. They chew on fences, barn doors, feed boxes, dirt, tree bark, bones and paint and a good farmer, rancher or husbandry man knows when a horse or cow cribs the animal really has a craving for nutritional minerals. A good husbandry man will give the animals minerals to save the animals life, to keep the veterinary bills down and to keep from having to rebuild the fence or barn – animals will literally eat the barn in their search for minerals. Such mineral starved animals will at first eat large amounts of supplemental minerals until they are satisfied, then they will automatically reduce their level of consumption to a maintenance level.

"Salt appetite" is very striking in both pregnant animals and humans. Bizarre cravings are legendary in the pregnant human. From antiquity, the description of cravings or pica in humans relates its major incidence to pregnant women.

The Hawaiian King Kamehameha's mother, Queen Kekuiapoiwa had cravings for eye-balls, although she specifically wanted chiefs eyes, she was given the eyes of sharks to eat.

We have seen a hundred pregnant Montana sheep lined up along a creek embankment eating the clay walls – this form of pica known as "geophagia" or earth -eating. Geophagia is very common among minerally deficient pregnant humans, especially women in the lower end of the economic scale – they will eat dirt from their yard. Geophagia is so common in the southeastern region of the United States that prepackaged clay is often sold in grocery stores in the dairy department.

Pica, or perverted appetite or irresistible cravings with the eating of bizarre or unsuitable nonfood substances (or fattening nonfoods) has been a curiosity for philosophers, doctors and priests for thousands of years. Pica as a symptom of mineral deficiencies is universal in the world and has been reported in animals and humans of all age groups. In modern times the easy availability of candy, sugared-high calorie snacks, soft drinks and junk foods has led to obesity when people feel the deep cravings of pica.

A doctoral thesis on pica by Agustus Fridericus Mergiletus (1701) begins with the definition of pica: " The malady pica is called "kitta" in Greek. Its derivation comes from the name of the common magpie because the bird ("pica" is the Latin name for magpie) itself is believed to suffer from some malady because it flits from tree to tree constantly seeking food or because it enjoys all sorts of foods."

A catalogue of bizarre instances of pica is found in Mergiletus' thesis. In men, he recorded one individual who ate leather, wood, nestlings and live mice. A second consumed woolen garments, leather, a live cat and some mice; a third ate cats' tales and decomposed human bodies with maggots!

In Mergiletus' female subjects he recorded women who ate human flesh including one particularly horrible lady – "she lured children with sweets, killed them and pickled them for her daily fare (sounds like a female version of Jeffrey Dahmer). The murders were only discovered when the woman's cat stole the pickled hand of a child and carried it over to the neighbors house."

The most common description of pica by Mergiletus were of women's desire for mud and mortar scrapped from walls (just like modern children who eat caulking and lead paint – we have often said that children who eat lead paint are screaming for minerals for their mineral-starved bodies – give them minerals and they won't eat lead paint); girls who ate their own hair; girls who ate cotton, thread from their own clothes, raw grain and lizards.

Mergiletus also described pica in animals including cats that ate wood ash and pregnant hunting dogs that ate unusual objects.

Cooper (1957) in her classic report on pica refers to several ancient and medieval writers who emphasized the occurrence of pica in pregnant women, i.e.- Aetios noted pregnant women to crave various and odd foods, some salty and some acid; some, he said "crave for sand, oyster shells and wood ashes." Aetios recommended a diet including "fruits, green vegetables, pigs feet, fresh fish and old tawny fragrant wine."

Boezo (1638) noted that pica occurred most often in pregnant women. Boezo saw pica as a physiological problem, and is the first to mention iron preparations as a treatment for pica – he suggested "one and one half scruples of iron dross taken for many days as wonderfully beneficial for men and women." Boezo also noted "the case of a virgin who was accustomed to devour salt in great quantities from which chronic behavior she developed diarrhea and wasting (Addisons Disease?)."

Christiani of Frankfurt (1691) reported a woman who ate 1,400 salt herrings during her pregnancy. LeConte (1846) suggested that animals eating earth do so because of "want of inorganic elements."

In modern times, the substances frequently reported as eaten as a result of pica behavior in humans includes paper, metallic gum wrappers, ice, dirt, coal, tar, clay, chalk, starch, baking powder, pebbles, wood, plaster, paint, chimney soot, hair, human and animal feces (kitty litter box) and cloth. Because of social constraints on our public behavior most people under public scrutiny who display pica eat sugar, snack food or smoke, drink alcohol or use street drugs (or prescription drugs) in an attempt to satisfy a nagging underlying craving.

Ice eating (pagophagia) is also common, especially for iron

deficient children and adults.

Worms have been reported as a cause of pica – Ankylostomiasis, ascariasis, oxyuriasis and others have been blamed. Parasites of course can cause anemia and malnutrition by direct blood sucking from the host or by competing for food in the gut. The anemia caused by parasitism is in fact perceived by the body as an iron deficiency anemia, which then results in the mineral craving behavior known as pica.

Dickens and Ford reported that 25% of all children ate earth. Cooper (1957) reported a 21% rate of pica in American Children referred to the Mothers Advisory Service in Baltimore.

Lanzkowsky (1959) reported that 12 children with pica had hemoglobin that ranged from 3 g% to 10.9 g% with a mean of 7.89 +/- 2.64. The institution of iron (i.m. – iron dextran) "resulted in a cure for pica in one to two weeks." It was demonstrated that calcium deficient weanling rats consume large amounts of a lead acetate solution (even though the solution tastes bad) when compared with calcium fed controls. Again, if children have sufficient nutritional minerals they will not eat lead paint.

McDonald and Marshall (1964) reported on 25 children who ate sand. They divided the group in half; they gave one of the two groups iron injections and the other group saline (salt solution). After three to four months 11 of the 13 children given iron had lost their pica behavior compared with only 3 of the 12 given saline.

Reynolds et al (1968) reported that 38 people with anemia exhibited pagophagia (ice eating) as the most common form of pica; 22 of 25 had their symptoms of pica disappear after correcting the iron depletion.

Woods and Weisinger (1970) reproduced pagophagia experimentally in rats by withdrawing blood. The pagophagia in the anemic rats was cured when the anemia was cured. It is of interest to note that pica or cribbing behaviors are not produced by vitamin deficiencies!

Two thirds of the 153 pregnant women studied by Taggart

(1961) developed cravings. The most common craving was for fruit, pickles, blood pudding, licorice, potato chips, cheese and kippers. A craving for sweets, vegetables, nuts and sweet pickles came in second place.

Phosphate appetite or phosphate cravings was described by LaVaillant (1796) as the anxious search by cattle in phosphate deficient South African pastures for discarded dog bones (osteophagia); they also chewed on wood (pica) and each other's horns. Bone chewing (osteophagia) has been reported in many wild species of herbivores including reindeer, caribou, red deer, camels, giraffe, elephant and wildebeest. We have seen elephants eating limestone roadbeds and large termite heaps as ready and available mineral supplements. The search for calcium rich edible clays and soils and territorial disputes over limited supplies by humans has led to endless wars in tribal Africa.

There is no evidence of a specific pica behavior for a magnesium supplement when laboratory animals are fed a magnesium deficient diet. Magnesium deficient animals will crave and eat common salt. Magnesium tastes bad enough that animals will die of magnesium deficiency initiated seizures rather than consume a pure magnesium supplement.

A natural potassium deficiency in humans is highly unlikely as all commonly consumed grains, fruits and vegetables, which tend to be rich in potassium. A potassium deficiency can be common in those individuals taking diuretics for high blood pressure, weight loss programs and starvation diets. Potassium deficient rats are hyperactive, hyper alert and lick everything including their metal cage, lab equipment, each other and urine puddles. It is of interest to note that even with a severe potassium deficiency laboratory rats have a strong craving for salt.

Chromium and vanadium deficiencies are manifested by extreme thirst for liquids (thirst is a common symptom of hypoglycemia and diabetes) with soft drinks being a frequent first choice and water the last.

The seven-food group pyramid fails to deal with the reality

that our American (and the worlds) food supply is deficient in essential minerals. If you want to make pigs fat give them carbohydrates. If you want to make cattle fat give them carbohydrates. If you want to make Americans fat give them the seven-food group pyramid!

Meal and snack portions constantly get larger both at home and at fast food and sit-down restaurants. An interesting survey showed that men ate 1.9 cups of pasta when served 2.5 cups of pasta; women consumed 1.4 cups when they were served 2.5 cups. Men consume 2.5 cups when they are served 5 cups of pasta; women consume 1.75 cups when they are served five cups. This means that people get 600 calories per "serving" of pasta today rather than the 200 calories of yesteryear!

A large serving of fries today is seven ounces compared to 2.4 ounces in a small serving of fries – this means 610 calories in the large serving versus 210 calories in the small serving!

A large four-ounce deli cookie contains 500 calories, whereas a standard half-ounce cookie contains only 60 calories. The 64-ounce soft drink contains 800 calories compared to 80 calories in the standard soft drink! Remember, Wallach's Law – mineral deficiencies produce cravings that result in obesity, optimal levels of dietary or supplemental minerals eliminates cravings which results in optimal weight loss and weight control.

Americans suffer from violence, rage, obesity, degenerative, fatal emotional and physical diseases resulting from specific nutritional mineral deficiencies. When the 90 essential nutrients are supplemented at the optimal levels in the proper form pica and cribbing in all their presentations are eliminated and weight loss and weight control are easily accomplished by anyone that makes a serious effort – Wallach's Law of weight loss and weight management is as predictable as gravity!

There are several basic dietary practices that can be added to Wallach's Law and the mineral supplement program to assure and speed up weight loss and guarantee weight control:

- Drink 8 – 10 glasses of water daily – as much as 40% of our daily water comes from our food. Cut back on calories and you cut back on water – thirst is often misinterpreted as hunger.
- No carbonated drinks – they neutralize stomach acid and then you can't efficiently absorb minerals, digest protein or absorb vitamin B12.
- No caffeine – caffeine (i.e.- coffee, iced tea, hot tea, soft drinks, chocolate, etc.) initially raises blood sugar and gives an energy hit – in an hour or so later the blood sugar drops precipitously causing a ravenous hunger.
- No carbohydrates – there are no nutritional requirements for carbohydrates – we easily make blood glucose from fats (this is what you want to happen) and proteins. Eat high quality animal proteins (i.e.- eggs, red meat, poultry, fish and whey); eat lots of green leafy vegetables, tomatoes, carrots, celery, etc.
- Employ Dr. Wallach's salad fork trick – never put salad dressing on your salad! The no-fat low calorie salad dressings still have 90 to 150 calories per tablespoon (10 tablespoons per salad could be 1,000 calories per salad!); never dip a fork full of salad into the salad dressing – the trick is to dip your salad fork vertically ¼ inch into a small bowl or shot glass of salad dressing (no scooping!). Dr. Wallach's salad fork trick will give you the taste of salad dressing with only 30 calories per salad!
- No eating after 7:00 pm – 85% of the weight gaining calories that are consumed in America, are consumed after dinner. Drink all the water you want after dinner but no calories – if you are hungry after 7:00 pm it means you didn't eat enough animal protein at dinner. If you are desperately hungry eat mixed salted nuts or a sugar free whey shake.
- GET RID OF THE MUNCHIES – supplement with all 90

essential nutrients; pay special attention to all 60 essential minerals in the plant derived colloidal form and the major minerals and the electrolytes in the chelated and ionic form to ensure optimal intake.

• Employ mild diuretic and mild laxative herbs to reduce water weight and impacted stool (this technique alone can result in the loss of inches and several pounds!).

• Employ fat burners that include pyruvate – the metabolic fuel that drive cellular metabolism (the more pyruvate, the faster your metabolism goes); amino acid concentrates that are designed to burn calories while you sleep; and chromium picolinate (legendary amongst body builders for burning fat from under the skin).

• Employ fat blockers that can include chitosan, a finely ground shrimp shell flour that blocks as much as 7,000 – 10,000 calories (almost totally from saturated fat) per week.

By employing the simple truth of Wallach's Law and mineral supplement program techniques you will be able to lose 15, 25, 50, 75, 100, 125, 150 or even 200 pounds and keep it off. Low carbohydrate diets alone won't do it; high protein diets alone won't do it. To be successful in losing weight and keeping it off requires dealing with the basic root cause of weight gain – mineral deficiencies! Remember Wallach's Law says, "When you are minerally deficient you will gain weight; when you supplement with minerals you will lose weight!"

Chapter 8

Medical Dogmas and Lies or Show me the money!

> *"Fifty three percent of medical doctors in America admit they lie to get paid for procedures that the patient didn't get or didn't need."*
>
> —Journal of the American Medical Association

Insurance companies want you to believe they are selling you "health insurance" – when in fact they are really selling "insurance to protect you from outrageous medical fees." State and federal governments buy votes by "selling" you Medicare and Medicaid, which protects you from outrageous medical fees. A 1999 AMA study revealed that more than 50% percent of licensed medical doctors in America admit they lie to get paid by insurance for procedures they didn't do or that the patient really didn't need.

According to the insurance industry watchdogs as much as 75% of private medical insurance fraud and Medicare fraud are perpetuated by medical doctors yet few if any are prosecuted. Fifty two billion dollars are fraudulently extracted from Medicare and private insurance companies by doctors annually as "a right" that doctors consider a victimless crime.

Stealing from private and government insurance companies is so easy that the mafia has infiltrated the insurance system. Unlike prostitution, gambling and illegal drugs there are few if any risks of prosecution and punishment if one is caught stealing from and defrauding private insurance, Medicare or Medicaid.

Doctors believe it is a good thing to control health care costs as long as the controls don't impact their income. As third party payers (insurance companies and Medicare) cut back on services and costs they will cover and pay for, doctors get more creative on how to steal from insurance companies and Medicare, which they believe is their personal cash reserves. Doctors believe that stealing from private insurance and Medicare is a victimless crime and therefore justifiable.

We would all like to believe that our doctors in America are altruistic and are in the medical field as a result of their love of people and their desire to help people who are sick and miserable; and that their accumulated wealth is an indirect reward for their good and kindly work. Unfortunately medicine is a business that gets paid whether you get better or not, it is a business that gets paid whether you live or die. Medical doctors are the "stock brokers" of health – they win when you're buying or selling; they win whether you're winning or losing and they win whether you live or die.

Once you realize that your doctor is more interested in your insurance number than your personal well being you will begin to understand the truth and you will be a little safer.

Thousands of people ask us each year, "If the nutritional approach to prevent and cure disease is proven and has few if any negative side effects, how come my doctor doesn't incorporate the information in our treatment program?" The answer is simple – there are no financial incentives for him to use them, it is not to his financial benefit to use them. Right or wrong is not a factor in the decision to not use nutritional approaches to preventing and curing disease.

There are no laws that require a doctor to cure you even if a cure is available! There are no laws that require a doctor to prevent disease in you even if a method of prevention is known. The only way to ensure your own maximum health and longevity is to read and educate yourself – you can save yourself an enormous amount of unnecessary misery, save yourself a gob of money and add 20, 30, 40 or 50 extra healthful years to your life by taking over the responsibility for your own health! Do not leave your success for health and longevity in the hands of a profession or trade that first says, "Show me the money!"

Pharmaceutical companies pay out $14 billion each year in "advertising," promotional giveaways and outright kickbacks to doctors to encourage them to prescribe their drugs. Doctors will boldly say to pharmaceutical detail reps, " I'd be happy to use your product if I can get a fishing trip to Cabo San Lucas out of the deal" or "I'll be happy to use your products if my lifetime country club membership is paid up" or "I'll be happy to use your product if a shiny new black Mercedes is in my driveway next week."

Isn't it funny how doctors believe animal research when it comes to pharmaceuticals and they get kickbacks to "believe" and they don't believe in animal research when it comes to nutritional approaches to preventing or curing disease because they don't get kickbacks or incentives to "believe."

Medical dogmas are lies that doctors will profess to be a medical fact. If they base their diagnosis, treatment plan and prescriptions for you on these medical dogmas the odds are you won't live to be 100 years of age, the odds are you will suffer from poly pharmacy and be sick and miserable over the last 15 to 20 years of your life.

Dr. Ma Lan and I know of at least 500 medical dogmas and lies that make humans miserable, turn us into slaves of the medical system and shorten the lifespan of Americans. The following are just a few of the major medical dogmas and lies. Knowing these medical dogmas and lies for what they are, knowing what to correctly do to protect ourselves from these outrages will free you from medical slavery, save you an enormous amount of unnecessary misery, save you a gob of money and add many healthful years to your life.

Exercise

There are sports medicine doctors, cardiologists, orthopedic surgeons, family practitioners, medical fitness experts, personal trainers and their followers who want you to believe that exercise, strength training and cardiovascular toning through aerobic exercise is the answer to health and longevity, yet few if any professional athletes, personal trainers or fitness experts have lived to be 100 years of age.

Exercise buffs eat the seven-food group pyramid and with the exception of body builders and weight lifters, athletes forego serious supplementation programs - if it's not in the seven-food group pyramid I don't need it!

Fortunately, we have the World Wildlife Fund, Green Peace and the American Humane Society to protect animal species and monitor, mourn or eulogize endangered or extinct species; yet, who will monitor, mourn and eulogize the flower of American youth – the high school, college, weekend and professional athlete?

Three young men, Reggie Lewis of the Boston Celtics (died July 28, 1993 at the age of 27); Hank Gathers of Loyola Marymount, Los Angeles, California (died in March 1990 at age 23); and Terry Cummings of the San Antonio Spurs (limited to 30 minutes of play by an irregular heart beat in 1983). All three highly visible and "healthy" young athletes died or were in serious physical trouble from cardiomyopathy (muscular dystrophy of the heart) – a simple deficiency of the trace mineral selenium.

Len Bias, a 1986 top draft choice of the Celtics, died from heart failure two days after he was selected. An autopsy showed the presence of cocaine, but was cocaine the cause of death?

Dr. George Sheehan, the late editor of Running World Magazine summed it up for most athletes - "I won't let food supplements or diets interfere with my running." Dr. Sheehan died at age 75 from prostate cancer.

Jim Fixx, the running guy who started the whole individual fitness craze for the average American in the 1970s died in 1982 at age 52 from his fifth heart attack – there is a serious problem with the theory that exercise is good for you and promotes health and longevity when the guru of personal fitness dies at age 52 from a heart attack!

Dr. James Cornyn was a cardiologist from Paradise, California, his wife is a cardiologist – they lived the idyllic low stress life exercising, jogging through the redwood forest, eating right and taking all of the medications he prescribed to his patients to thin their blood, lower cholesterol, avoiding bad foods and exercising - yet he died at age 48 from a heart attack. If you were one of his heart patients would you keep on doing what he recommended that you do? I wouldn't, I would do just the opposite of whatever he said to do because I wouldn't want to get what he got.

If doctor Cornyn said to exercise 30 minutes per day I would not exercise at all; if he said to avoid eggs I would eat 25 per day; if he said no butter I would eat a stick of butter for dessert every day because I wouldn't want to get what he got!

After a serious search we can't find a single professional athlete of a major sport who has lived to be a centenarian (Table 2-1)! In fact the more talented the athlete, the more they participate in their sport the more likely they are to die young.

Table 2-1. Athlete's death age, sport and cause.

Name	Sport	Cause	Age
Red Grange	football	Parkinson's Disease	88
Jesse Owens	track	cancer	66
Jim Thorpe	football	heart attack	65
Babe Ruth	baseball	cancer	53

Lou Gehrig	baseball	ALS	38
Wilma Rudolph	track	brain tumor	54
Babe Zaharias	golf	breast cancer	43
Jim Fixx	track	heart attack	52
Hank Gathers	basketball	cardiomyopathy	23
Wilt Chamberlain	basketball	congestive heart failure	63
Reggie Lewis	basketball	cardiomyopathy	27
Walter Payton	football	liver disease	45
S. Grenkoff	figure skating	cardiomyopathy	28
Flojo	track	"seizure"	35
Don Drysdale	baseball	heart attack	56
Kory Stringer	football	"heat stroke"	27

The average couch potato in America not only outlives American family practitioners but they also outlive the average American professional athlete!

Professional athletes start training and participating in sports in a regimented fashion by the time they are six years old – pee-wee soccer, pee-wee hockey, pee-wee softball, pee-wee baseball, gymnastics, basketball, golf, tennis, etc.

According to the CDC 100,000 young Americans under the age of 30 drop dead each year during or immediately following exercise or a game and that 300,000 Americans over the age of 30 drop dead annually during or after exercise. We have a problem with the theory that exercise in of itself is good for you. Another dogmatic "health truth," another medical dogma fails the test of time.

The basic problem with exercise lies in the fact that athletes sweat more in five years than couch potatoes sweat in 75 years. The same concern regarding sweat holds true for farmers, ranchers, roofers, carpenters, electricians, plumbers, carpet layers, dance instructors, bakers and office workers who go to health clubs and sweat.

Sweat is not only composed of water, sweat is not just laden with salt. Sweat is a complex soup that contains all of the nutritional components found in blood - all essential nutrients. The very act of sweating is a sudden drain on ones levels of circulating blood nutrients and a chronic drain on our deep nutrient reserves and without a constant replacement of this loss of nutrients is to invite disaster.

Drinking water alone does not replace the essential nutrients normally found in sweat; drinking traditional electrolyte (salt) and sugar laden sports drinks does not replace the essential nutrients found in sweat; carbonated water and soft drinks do not replace the essential nutrients found in sweat; neither coffee nor iced tea will replace the essential nutrients lost in sweat and all have additional long term dangers associated with them including dehydration and nutrient absorption problems.

Carbonated drinks neutralize stomach acid, which significantly reduces the absorption efficiency of minerals, the ability to digest proteins (pepsin won't work in a neutral or alkaline environment) and the absorption of vitamin B12 (intrinsic factor, necessary for the absorption of vitamin B12 won't work in a neutral or alkaline environment).

In a June 2000 Harvard study of 460 female teenage athletes one non-cola carbonated drink per day increased the risk of fractures and osteoporosis over water drinkers by as much as 300%, while the consumption of cola carbonated drinks increases the risk of fractures and osteoporosis over water drinkers by as much as 500%!

Injury, degenerative disease and early death are the inheritance of serious athletes who do not pay attention to their body's micronutrient nutritional needs. Trainers teach and preach strength training as the way to reduce risks of injury. Athletes seem to willingly accept these statistics of personal doom in exchange for a short "good life" of fame and fortune. We have lectured to professional, university and Olympic level athletes and we find that the athlete's willingness to spread the truth about the need to replace micronutrients lost in sweat can't compete with the promise of royalties for testimonies and giveaways for high performance athletes.

This terrible injury and life-threatening negative that faces athletes every day they practice or participate in an event can be counteracted and eliminated by total replacement of all nutrients lost in sweat.

The bottom line is that we don't need to be an athlete to sweat! You can be a farmer, rancher, roofer, carpenter, electrician, plumber, carpet layer, bakery worker, dance instructor or harried single mother of three and sweat. Replacement of the nutrients that are sweat out during exercise or labor will save you an enormous amount of unnecessary misery, add many healthful years to your life and save you a gob of money.

Cardiovascular Disease

Heart or cardiovascular diseases are listed as the number one cause of death in Americans yet cardiovascular disease is not a single "disease" - cardiovascular diseases are a collection of nutritional deficiency diseases that affect the cardiovascular system. Contrary to the popular medical marketing hype there is no cardiovascular disease that is genetically transmitted or caused by elevated blood levels of cholesterol or triglycerides.

Doctors want you to believe that the genesis or cause of all cardiovascular disease is directly or indirectly (genetically) related to blood cholesterol levels – this is absolutely absurd and untrue! Doctors have made Americans so paranoid about cholesterol levels that in 1998 Americans were willing to spend between $117 and $158 billion annually for cholesterol testing alone, by comparison Americans spent only $185 billion for their military defense in 1998.

We have known for 75 years in the animal industry that cholesterol is not the "bogey-man" that medical doctors would have you believe it is. Can you ever recall a veterinarian getting excited about your dog, cat, bird, fish or livestock's blood cholesterol? Of course not! Elevated blood cholesterol or elevated blood triglycerides do not cause a single disease – they are in fact warning signals for other problems (i.e.- hypothyroidism, diabetes, deficiencies of niacin, chromium, vanadium, essential fatty acids, liver disease, etc.).

Doctors want Americans to get their blood cholesterol below 200 while according to Dr. Steven B. Hulley from the University of California, San Francisco 220 to 270 is the normal range for humans. Red meat and eggs have no more effect on raising blood cholesterol than chicken and fish. In fact the more eggs you eat the lower your cholesterol will go – even the American Heart Association says that eating two eggs each day is safe and even encouraged as a source of high quality proteins and luteins.

Luteins are cousins to beta-carotene that clean cholesterol from your arteries. The more eggs you eat the cleaner your arteries will be – just don't fry them or cook them in margarine.

The Eskimos above the Arctic Circle have a traditional diet that is 98% red meat and blubber (i.e.- whale meat, whale blubber, walrus meat, walrus blubber, seal meat, seal blubber, bear meat, bear fat, salmon, etc.) – not a single Eskimo has a juicer or eats organically grown vegetables, their blood cholesterols range from 250 – 350 and yet they are legendary for not getting cardiovascular disease.

The truth is that cardiovascular disease is a collection of diseases caused by a variety of nutritional deficiencies and just lowering blood cholesterol levels below 200 does not reduce the risk of any disease any more than reducing the number of weather reports will reduce the number of tornadoes and there is significant evidence to show that low cholesterol levels (below 200) increases ones risk of stroke, cerebral hemorrhage, liver cancer, chronic obstructive pulmonary disease, Alzheimer's disease and depression resulting in suicide by 200 to 300%!

Stroke
Blood clot (thrombosis) – essential fatty acid deficiency
Ruptured aneurysm – copper deficiency

Anemia – deficiency of any one of the 90 essential nutrients, although iron, copper, selenium, calcium, folic acid, vitamin E, vitamin C and vitamin B12 deficiencies are most common.

Coronary thrombosis – deficiency of any one of the essential fatty acids, magnesium and manganese.

Arteriosclerosis – magnesium deficiency, selenium deficiency, lutein deficiency, folic acid deficiency, vitamin C deficiency.

Cardiomyopathy – heart disease – selenium deficiency, vitamin E deficiency, methionine deficiency.

Congestive heart failure – vitamin B1 deficiency (wet beri – beri); selenium deficiency (hypertrophic cardiomyopathy).

Prolapsed mitral valve – magnesium deficiency

Atrial fibrillation – osteoporosis, magnesium deficiency, selenium deficiency

Aneurysm – copper deficiency

Varicose veins (hemorrhoids) – copper deficiency

Pharmaceuticals and invasive procedures may be useful on occasion for stabilizing catastrophic emergency cardiovascular events, however, most cardiovascular disease is preventable and correctable with simple nutritional supplement programs. We also know that if angioplasty is necessary that serious supplementation with folic acid (vitamin B9), pyradoxene (vitamin B6) and cyanocobalamine (vitamin B12) will reduce re-stenosis by as much as 48%.

Diabetes

Diabetes is being diagnosed in epidemic numbers in America – a million new cases each year. There are 32 million diabetics in the United States or fully 12% of the nearly 300 million Americans. Adult onset type II diabetics make up 95% or 29 million of the diabetic population – they make more insulin than non-diabetics, sometimes as much as 10 times more insulin than non-diabetics. Type I or juvenile onset diabetics do not make any insulin.

The differential diagnosis of type II or type I diabetes used to be easy, one could simply diagnose it by age of onset – under the age of 12 years - type I; over the age 45 years- type II. These historically well-demarcated age differences between type I diabetes and type II diabetes have now merged together and cannot be diagnosed simply by age of onset. The diagnosis of type II diabetes has soared in Americans in their 30s; the age group that has the most rapid increase in rate of diagnosis of type II diabetes are kids under the age of twelve.

There is currently an epidemic of new diabetes cases in America – one million new cases per year! There are two reasons for this epidemic - a significant increase in America's intake of sugar and carbohydrates and a rapid fall in the intake of the mineral cofactors necessary (i.e. – chromium and vanadium) for insulin to function properly.

In 1948 the level of chromium in American blood was 28 mcg/L today it is 0.13 mcg/L. Drastic drops in soil levels of chromium and vanadium and the almost exclusive use of processed white flower in breads and pasta has all but eliminated optimal levels of chromium and vanadium from American food supplies – the only way to guarantee enough chromium and vanadium in the American diet to prevent and reverse hypoglycemia and all of its manifestations (i.e.- ADD, ADHD, panic attacks, anxiety attacks, rage, depression, manic depression, bipolar diseases), narcolepsy (hyperinsulinemia) and adult onset type II diabetes is to supplement daily with optimal levels of chromium and vanadium.

According to the USDA in 1895 Americans were eating about ½ pound of sugar per person per year, this increased steadily to 157 pounds of sugar per person per year (almost a half a pound each day) by 1999. This huge increase in American sugar consumption reflects an almost total dependence on boxed, packaged, bottled and canned foods – especially soft drinks, juices, candy and cold cereals. The acceptance of this much sugar in the American diet is also a reflection of mineral deficiencies and the resultant pica behavior and a craving for sweets or salt.

A 2002 Harvard School of Public Health study of 42,504 men between the ages of 40 and 75 showed that men who frequently eat hot dogs, bacon, sausage and other sugar containing processed meats are 46% more likely to develop type II diabetes than men who eat less of the food. The big increase in risk came among men who ate the processed meats five times or more each week. "This effect is dose related – the more you eat of these foods, the higher the risk," says Frank Hu, senior author of the study.

Adult onset type II diabetes is a simple mineral deficiency disease that was eliminated as a disease in laboratory and pet animals fed complete dietary formulas as early as 1957. Complete chromium and vanadium supplement programs employed in humans based on these animal formulas have been extremely successful in lowering blood sugar levels and reducing the need for or even totally wean off of insulin and other diabetes medication. One must take and record their blood sugar levels each morning and their medicine (insulin or pills) levels must be adjusted to prevent insulin shock – remember adult onset type II diabetics make lots of insulin!

If the fact that adult onset type II diabetes was known to be a simple mineral deficiency disease since 1957 when Dr. Walter Mertz published his landmark PhD thesis in Federation Proceedings, the official journal of the National Institute of Health - how come your doctor has not told you?

The GAO says that each diabetic over the 25 to 40 years they live after diagnosis is worth to their doctors between $600,000 to $750,000 – how many doctors do you know who are honest enough to give up $750,000 to tell you the truth?

Iron deficiency anemia is treated with iron supplements (no money here) while adult onset diabetes type II (a deficiency disease of chromium and vanadium) and its complications are treated with amputations of toes, feet and legs, kidney dialysis, kidney transplant, angiograms, angioplasty, stints, coronary by-pass surgery, heart transplant, lowering cholesterol, laser treatment of detached retinas, cataract surgery, peripheral neuropathies and prescriptions for high blood pressure – lots of money here! Cha-ching! Cha-ching!

Arthritis/Osteoporosis

Osteoporosis and arthritis are not genetically transmitted. Osteoporosis and arthritis are really a collection of multiple mineral and nutrient deficiencies. While primarily a calcium deficiency problem, these 147 different calcium deficiency diseases collectively known as osteoporosis and arthritis have a more complicated etiology and pathogenesis than just a simple calcium deficiency.

Osteoporosis and arthritis strikes both sexes equally! A five year Canadian study on 10,000 participants from nine centers showed that men are equally susceptible to hip fractures, compression fractures and systemic osteoporosis and osteoarthritis as women. The study, published in November 2001 involved x-rays and bone density scans in 3,000 men and 6,000 women over the age of 50, showed that 25% of the men had clinical osteoporosis and arthritis – the same percentage of osteoporosis as the women.

Medical dogma prior to this 2001 Canadian study falsely trumpeted that only post-menopausal women were in serious danger of osteoporosis and its complications. This Canadian study reiterates the fact that osteoporosis in women and men is a simple mineral deficiency disease and has nothing to do with a post-menopausal dip in estrogen production.

Studies have shown that women receiving estrogen therapy or HRT do not preserve bone mass any more efficiently than women receiving sugar pills.

The mineral analysis of normal animal and human bones contain more than 60 different minerals and a rubbery tendon-like material that acts as a frame work or lattice to accept minerals in an organized fashion resulting in what we call bone – you can not lay down new minerals in growing or depleted bones without first laying down new bone matrix.

Doctors have the criminal belief that your bones are nothing but a pile of calcium or worse yet TUMS – no wonder they "can't rebuild lost bone mass after the age of 50."

A simple "Mr. Wizard" home experiment will prove to you that this belief that bones are only a pile of calcium is false. First eat the meat off of two chicken drumstick bones, clean them up so they are free of meat scraps; hold one by the ends and attempt to bend it into a horseshoe shape – it will not bend but rather will snap like a dry twig; the second cleaned up chicken drumstick bone place into a quart of distilled vinegar for a month – after removing the chicken bone from the vinegar you will immediately notice that something dramatic has happened, the bone is now a floppy wet noodle because most of the minerals have been leeched from the bone by the vinegar leaving only the bone matrix. The bone matrix looks like the chicken drumstick bone but contains little or no minerals and is subject to compression fractures.

Bones afflicted with osteoporosis are not really brittle but rather they are rubbery and will fold and kink producing what is known as compression fractures of the vertebrae and long bones as a result of the pressures of normal weight bearing and simple daily activities.

Many dietary habits and medicine intakes (prescription or over the counter) interfere with the absorption, utilization and storage of nutrients including minerals. High fiber diets contain phytates that create mineral/phytate complexes that can not be absorbed, high fat diets that combine with minerals to form soap, carbonated drinks that neutralize stomach acid and reduce your ability to absorb minerals digest protein and absorb vitamin B12, phosphates (soft drinks, high protein diets – plant and animal) increase the dietary need for calcium and high caffeine consumption (500 mg/day) from tea, coffee and soft drinks that dump minerals from body stores are serious problems that can increase the rate of mineral deficiency diseases by as much as 500%.

Medications such as Prednazone, cortisone, anti-seizure drugs and diuretics and kidney dialysis are legendary for depletion of mineral reserves and increasing the rate of lose of stored minerals especially calcium, magnesium and potassium.

As bones lose minerals for any reason and blood levels of calcium drop they respond to increased blood levels of the parathyroid gland hormone, parathormone, which causes an increased rate of connective tissue or bone matrix production (remember the chicken drumstick bone experiment). Extremes of this process result in osteoporosis (147 different diseases), osteoarthritis, degenerative arthritis, ankylosing spondylitis of vertebrae, peripheral neuropathies, periodontal disease, bone spurs, heel spurs, calcium deposits, Osgood – Schlauter disease, kidney stones, fibrous osteodystrophy, compression fractures, myelofibrosis (filling of bone marrow cavity with bone matrix), Paget's disease, etc.

There are 12 pairs of cranial nerves and 31 pairs of spinal nerves (86 peripheral nerves in all) that have a potential for being pinched or crushed as they exit the brain and spinal cord through or between bones. These pinched or crushed nerves produce peripheral neuropathy diseases such as optic neuralgia, trigeminal neuralgia, Bell's palsy, tinnitis, deafness, Wallach's vertigo, pseudoangina, atrial fibrillation, sciatica, spinal stenosis, burning or numb feet, etc.

As bones generate significant and excessive amounts of the fibrous connective tissue it begins to impinge on nerves passing through canals and foramen found between and through individual bones resulting in commonly recognized peripheral neuropathies. Peripheral neuropathies are nothing more than a predictable complication of osteoporosis and the excess connective tissue generated as a result of a high output of parathormone by the hyperactive parathyroid glands.

In addition to thickening bones (Paget's disease) and filling canals and foramen (peripheral neuropathies), the connective tissue generated as a result of osteoporosis also fills the bone marrow cavity squeezing and choking off the cells that generate red blood cells, white blood cells and platelets (myelofibrosis).
Initially myelofibrosis is symptom free, however, as the connective tissue builds up in the bone marrow cavity anemia, fatigue, weight loss and malaise appear. The false medical belief is that Paget's disease and myelofibrosis are autoimmune diseases that are incurable and eventually fatal despite the very best of medical treatment (transfusions, cortisone and chemotherapy).

Contrary to popular medical belief, Paget's disease and myelofibrosis are nothing more than advanced stages of and variations on osteoporosis known as nutritional secondary hyperparathyroidism (NSH) or fibrous osteodystrophy – easily prevented and easily reversed with nutritional osteoporosis re-architecturing programs.

In spite of considerable medical effort and thought, the global etiology and pathogenesis of bone disease including cranial and spinal peripheral neuropathies, has not been "discovered" by the orthodox medical community and as a result there are no generally accepted universal orthodox therapies because the medical and pharmaceutical industries are busy searching for drugs that can be patented.

There are 12 pairs (24) of cranial nerves, each arising from a cellular "nucleus" in the brain and then each exiting the skull via a canal or foramen. The compression of any of the 24 cranial nerves results in unilateral motor or sensory neuropathies (Table 1). Historically approximately 10 percent of cranial neuropathies could be attributed to a specific etiology (i.e.- trauma, tumor, abscess, viral infections, Herpes zoster, multiple sclerosis, demyelinating diseases, aneurysms, etc.) the remaining 90 percent were dubbed by orthodox doctors as idiopathic or cause unknown.

Because cranial nerves exit the skull via a canal or foramen, any reduction in caliber of the foramen or canal has the potential for partial or complete strangulation of the nerve. The 24 bones of the skull, face and jawbone are equally victimized by systemic diseases of the skeleton (i.e.- osteoarthritis, osteoporosis, fibrous osteodystrophy, Paget's disease, NSH, etc.). The remainder of the bones of the skeleton -vertebrae, ribs, long bones, digits and flat bones (skull, facial bones, jaw bone, pelvis, etc.) are not the only bones affected by mineral deficiencies.

Table 1. Cranial Neuropathies and the Affected Cranial Nerve

Nerve	Disorder
I (Olfactory)	loss of the sense of smell

II (Optic)	optic nerve neuropathy, anopsia, blindness.
III (Occulomotor)	Horner's syndrome, diplopia, unevenly dilated pupils, ptosis, lateral eye diviation
IV (Trochlear)	double vision
V (Trigeminal)	trigeminal neuralgia
VI (Abducens)	inability to look toward side of 6th cranial nerve strangulation
VII (Facial)	Bell's palsy, Sjogren's disease (dry eyes), loss of taste ant. 2/3 of tongue.
VIII(Vestibulcochlear)	tinnitis, Wallach's vertigo (formerly Meinere's dx), deafness
IX (Glossopharyngeal)	pain in pharynx, low blood pressure
X (Vagus)	hoarseness, loss of gag reflex, can't swallow, hiccups
XI (Spinal accessory)	wasting of neck, can't shrug shoulder, wry neck (cervical dystonia)
XII (Hypoglossal)	wasting of tongue, deviation to side

Classical medical approaches to treating cranial neuropathies included surgery, antiviral, analgesic and anti-inflammatory pharmaceuticals, which typically have negative systemic side effects (i.e.- osteoporosis, arthritis, etc.) and these approaches fail to have a positive and lasting effect because the basic disease process has not been dealt with.

In contrast to the general lack of understanding of the etiology and pathogenesis of cranial peripheral neuropathies there is considerable understanding of the etiology and pathogenesis of spinal peripheral neuropathies. There are 31 pairs (62) of spinal nerves, each arising from motor or sensory cellular "nucleus" in the brain or spinal cord and then each exiting the spinal canal via a "canal" or notch formed by grooves between neighboring vertebrae. The compression of any of the 62 spinal nerves results in unilateral or bilateral motor or sensory "peripheral" neuropathies (Table 2).

Table 2. Spinal Peripheral Neuropathies Caused by Incarcerated Nerves

Psuedoangina

Tachycardia   (fast heart beat)

Bradycardia   (slow heart beat)

Atrial fibrillation   (palpitations; aryhthmia)

Hiccups

Hypochlorhydria   (lack of stomach acid)

"gallbladder" attacks   (pain in the upper right quadrant of abdomen)

Reflex sympathetic dystrophy   (RSD - chronic regional pain following a neck or spinal injury)

Spinal stenosis

"Post polio syndrome"   (wasting of one or both legs)

Sciatica   (pain, numbness, burning, itching of feet, legs and buttocks)

Peripheral neuropathy   (arms/legs/feet)

Restless leg syndrome

Constipation

Diarrhea

Urinary incontinence

Urinary retention

Impotence

Almost 100 percent of non-traumatic spinal peripheral neu-ropathies are attributable to nerve compression as a result of shrinking inter-vertebral disc, bone spurs, calcium deposits, osteoarthritis, degenerative arthritis, ankylosing spondylitis of the vertebrae, fibrous osteodystrophy, nutritional secondary hyper-parathyroidism and osteoporosis.

The reduction in the percentage of mineral density in any bone results in the overproduction of bone matrix, a rubbery ten-don-like material – it appears to be this fibrous connective tissue that reduces the caliber of cranial foramen and canals and com-presses cranial nerves producing the cranial neuropathy.

The consumption of carbonated drinks, high fiber diets (phy-tates), caffeine and sugar exacerbates a calcium deficiency by reducing absorption, utilization and retention efficiency and thereby indirectly stimulating the parathyroid gland to extract excessive calcium from bone reserves.

Blood glucose pathology has been shown to specifically increase the risk of deafness, Wallach's vertigo, and tinnitis. One study of 1,400 patients with inner ear symptoms including Wallach's vertigo, most had blood sugar problems including diabetes. In these cases the correction of blood sugar levels, elimination of sugar consumption and the correction of calcium deficiency eliminates the symptoms of the peripheral neuropathy disease. Another study showed that 75 per cent of 50 Wallach's vertigo patients had abnormal blood glucose tests.

Blood calcium levels associated with any of the cranial or spinal neuropathies may be low normal, below normal or even elevated (nutritional secondary hyperparathyroidism or fibrous osteodystrophy).

The more commonly occurring cranial nerve neuropathies (i.e.- optic neuralgia, Bell's palsy, trigeminal neuralgia, tinnitis, Wallach's vertigo, etc.) occur at a higher rate than the others because of the snug fit of a large firm nerve passing through a relatively small caliber canal or foramen – thus any bone pathology that produces an increase in bone connective tissue will trigger one or more different neuropathies by reducing the caliber of the canal or foramen.

The nutritional rebuilding and re-architecturing of bone pathology back to normal anatomy is well documented in both animals and humans. The bone rebuilding and re-architecturing process is equally effective for all bones of the body including the 24 bones of the skull (cranium and face) and jaw.

Women in their child bearing years are affected with Bell's palsy (BP) two to four times more often than men of the same age, and pregnant women 3.3 times more often than non-pregnant women. The majority of the BP of pregnancy occurs in the third trimester of pregnancy when the calcium needs of the fetus are the greatest.

The onset of the BP of pregnancy is sudden and painful – the supplemental use of prenatal vitamins and calcium result in a rapid and complete postnatal recovery for the mother and results in the neonatal outcome to be unaffected. The BP of pregnancy is a predictor of pre-eclampsia, gestational hypertension and toxemia – all of which are resolved quickly with high protein low sugar diets that are supplemented with adequate levels of calcium and magnesium.

Treat peripheral neuropathies nutritionally as you would osteoporosis and they simply go away!

Cancer

Cancer is not a genetically transmitted disease, less than 10% of cancers have anything remotely to do with genetics and according to a July 2000 report from the Karolynska Institute in Stockholm, Sweden, mapping out the human genome will not result in a cure for cancer. There are more lies told to the American public about cancer than any other disease – not too surprising, because there is more money involved with cancer than any other disease.

Low fat diets do not protect against cancer or lower your risk of getting it – the results of the Harvard Nurses Health Study (90,000 nurses over 20 years) showed that it doesn't matter whether you eat a diet containing 50% of your calories as fat or less than 20% of your calories as fat - there is no measurable decrease in cancer risk regardless of the amount of fat in your diet.

Cancer risk for breast, prostate and colon cancer can be raised by as much as 462 percent by eating burnt animal fat (butter, lard, suet, fried, well done meat, etc.) or hetero cyclic amines – it is not the amount of fat in your diet that is dangerous, but rather how you cook the fat that is dangerous!

It does not matter if you eat a diet high in fiber, as high fiber diets will not measurably lower your risk of colon or rectal cancer. The Harvard Nurses Health Study looked at 90,000 nurses and 50,000 male doctors (140,000 human subjects) over 20 years and demonstrated very clearly that high fiber diets do not measurably reduce the risk of cancer.

In fact the daily consumption of high fiber diets are risky as they can increase your risk of mineral deficiency diseases because of the phytate content. Phytates are carbon-phosphate compounds associated with plant fiber. Phytates form mineral/phytate complexes that can't be efficiently absorbed resulting in increased risk of arthritis, ankylosing spondylitis, osteoporosis, high blood pressure, cardiomyopathy heart disease, diabetes, lupus, bone spurs, kidney stones, loose teeth, periodontal disease, etc.

Multi-grain breads, raw vegetables and bran supplements are safe to eat two or three times a week but not two or three times a day! Steamed vegetables are safer than raw vegetables because the phytates found in raw vegetables are destroyed by heat. Juicers that remove and separate the juice from the fiber and pulp are safer than un-seperated vegetable juices.

Lastly it doesn't matter if you eat four to six servings of fruit and vegetables a day - they won't reduce your risk of cancer by any measurable amount! The Journal of the National Cancer Institute in November 2000 published a Harvard Nurses Health Study report on 136,000 health professionals over 16 years that showed four to six servings of fruit and vegetables a day reduces the risk of heart disease and diabetes but had zero effect in protecting you against colon and rectal cancer.

Cancer is caused by contact with bad substances (i.e.- foods, cooked or burnt food byproducts such as trans fatty acids and heterocyclic amines, tobacco, alcohol, industrial chemicals, agricultural chemicals, pharmaceuticals, etc.) and a failure to consume protectants such as antioxidants (selenium, vitamin E, vitamin A, vitamin C), flavonoids, catechins (EGCGs) and anti-angiogenic substances (shark cartilage, green tea, etc.) – paying special attention to consume and supplement with all of the good things daily and avoiding all of the bad things you can reduce your risk of cancer to almost zero!

The catechins or EGCGs found in green tea are reported to be 100 times more potent than vitamin C and 25 times more potent than vitamin E in neutralizing free radicals and in a Case Western Reserve University Medical School study, catechins from green tea reduced the risk of cancer in lab animals by 90 percent.

An English study showed that the optimal blood levels, of the trace mineral gallium in pregnant women, significantly reduces the risk of brain cancer in children. A 2002 study showed that more than five servings of processed meats per week can significantly increase the risk of brain cancer - the increase risk for brain cancer is dose related.

According to the Memorial Sloan Kettering Cancer Center in New York, arsenic trioxide can, at doses of 0.02 to 0.06 mg, put 11 of 12 acute promyelocytic leukemia patients into remission after only 30 days of supplementation and eight of the original 12 were still disease free a year latter. The original Chinese study showed acute promyelocytic leukemia patients were still disease free 10 years after starting the arsenic therapy!

The use of the trace mineral selenium to prevent and treat cancer is not a new concept – selenium was first reported as a cancer preventative and treatment in laboratory animals by a Professor Von Wasserman in April 1912!

More recently, studies by the University of California, San Diego (1980s), the National Cancer Institute (1993) and the University of Arizona School of Medicine (1996) demonstrated a significant anti cancer benefit in humans from supplementing with the trace mineral selenium, reducing all diseases by nine percent, stomach cancer by 21%, esophageal cancer by 71%, prostate cancer by 69%, colon cancer by 64%, lung cancer by 48% and breast cancer (depending on the type) by 65 to 85%.

"Curing" cancer will be a long, expensive, painful and perhaps a failed dream, while the prevention and long-term nutritional management (i.e.- antioxidants, anti-angiogenic substances, etc.) of cancer is simple, inexpensive, effective and available now as we speak! Avoid the bad things and consume the good things and you can reduce your risk of cancer by as much as 48% to 462%. If you already have cancer avoid the bad things and consume the good things and you can double or triple your predicted lifespan.

Alzheimer's disease

Alzheimer's disease is not a genetically transmitted disease. In July 1992 a joint report issued by the Salk Institute, famous for the polio vaccine and the University of California, San Diego school of Medicine that announced that large doses (2,000 IU) of vitamin E could help advanced Alzheimer's disease patients get back a significant amount of their memory. This UCSD study, considered an aberration by many investigators, was repeated and confirmed again in April 1997. Again the UCSD study showed that large doses of vitamin E given to advanced Alzheimer's patients could significantly delay the need for nursing home care. The simple use of vitamin E could save affected families as much as $500,000 – how many families received a postcard or letter from their medical doctor telling them the benefits of the use of vitamin E for their Alzheimer's affected spouse or parent?

In March of 1996 the Johns Hopkins University School of Medicine, based on a 14 year study of 2,000 seniors, announced that small daily doses of Ibuprofen can reduce your risk of Alzheimer's disease by as much as 60 percent. A November 2001 Dutch study showed an 80 percent reduction in risk of Alzheimer's disease in 7,000 seniors with the regular use of Ibuprofen.

A six year Dutch study of 5,395 people released in January of 2002 showed that three to five alcoholic drinks per day reduced the risk of Alzheimer's disease by 42 percent.

The blood enzyme homocystine, has been found to be consistently elevated in Alzheimer's patients. Homocystine levels can be brought back to normal levels within days by supplementation with large doses of folic acid.

High doses of the OTC NSAID Ibuprofen reversed as much as 30 percent of Alzheimer's plaque in just three days in laboratory animals.

The veterinary industry eliminated Alzheimer's disease (encephalomalacia) in animals more than 50 years ago using simple nutritional formulas with the right mix of essential fatty acids, dietary cholesterol and antioxidants (i.e.- vitamin E, selenium, etc.).

Alzheimer's disease is a simple nutritional deficiency disease created by the criminal advice of American medical doctors who are paranoid about fat and cholesterol. Over the past 50 years doctors have created a new class of diseases - cholesterol deficiency diseases – the worst of which is Alzheimer's disease. Alzheimer's disease was not recognized as a disease entity in America more than 40 years ago, even by another name it just didn't exist. Alzheimer's disease only became recognized as a disease entity in America after 1979 when it first began to appear in medical journals and textbooks.

Today, Alzheimer's disease is rated by some surveys as the number four killer of Americans over the age of 65 behind cardiovascular disease, cancer and diabetes – between the years 2000 and 2025 experts project 14 million Americans are going to die from this physician-caused cholesterol and antioxidant deficiency disease.

The brain contains a fatty insulating material (myelin) that coats and separates each nerve fiber. Myelin makes up 75% of the brain weight and myelin is almost 100% cholesterol – you can only manufacture about 10% of your daily need for cholesterol the other 90% must come from your diet.

Alzheimer's disease is easy to diagnose in brain tissue because much of the myelin disappears and the naked nerve fibers become tangled and look just like a "back lash" in your fishing reel.

If you are very, very good at following your doctors instructions and giving up butter and other dairy products, eggs, red meat and chicken skin guess what you are going to get – yep, you got it! Alzheimer's disease!

You do not want to give up natural sources of fat and cholesterol from your diet, just don't fry them or cook them in margarine! Supplement with all 90 essential nutrients and protect your brain from trans fatty acids and heterocyclic amine free radical damage – cholesterol for the brain is kind of like using a sunscreen on your skin to protect against skin cancer.

Mark our words, cholesterol will eventually officially be listed as an essential nutrient like vitamin A, vitamin C, calcium, zinc, amino acids and essential fatty acids in the next few years.

One must always remember that most of what doctors tell you about disease and nutrition (medical dogmas and lies) is at best misinformation passed along by the ignorant, and at the worst doctors pass on self serving information provided by pharmaceutical representatives who make their living by selling drugs to doctors; but since American doctors are informed of such things one can only class this misinformation as criminal fraud. Because doctors believe themselves omnipotent and think they are immortal they oftentimes have little or no common sense and as a result have an average lifespan of only 56 – 62 years depending on whose studies you believe.

If doctors were the holders of all medical truth and they practiced what they preached they should live longer and be healthier than the average American, however, the scorecard says doctors would rather continue to die young than to inform and educate themselves and their patients as to the value of nutritional supplementation!

There are no laws that say that doctors are required to prevent disease or cure patients even when there is a prevention or cure available! Remember, "Dead Doctors Don't Lie!" and "Live Doctors Do Lie!"

Chapter 9

The Epiphany

"Chance favors only the prepared mind."

—Louis Pasteur

*"Don't let your schooling get in the way
of your education"*

—Mark Twain

Missouri's mixed woods, great rivers, creeks, pastures and fields are a wonderland in the spring, summer, fall and winter. The spring Missouri air is warm and balmy; the March and April spring rains are soft and warm; and before the new oak leaves begin to burst from their buds the red bud and dogwood trees are in full bloom giving color to the dank woods.

The spring woods smell of wet moss and leaves; squirrels are prospecting in the leaves and probing the woodpecker holes in tree bark looking for their previously hidden acorn caches, birds are building nests and farmers are beginning the spring field preparation and planting – the earth was waking up from her winters sleep. It was the time to plant the tomato and bell pepper starts in the garden and plant the radish, squash, peas, beans and okra seeds; it was time to gather herbs and mushrooms. Dandelion greens and flowers collected from the yard and woods were used in salads and the tough yellow root was dried, cut into small shavings and steeped for a spring tonic.

The black Missouri gumbo bottomland soil is high in organic matter and its fertile musky smell fills the air as it is worked and turned. Snow-white cattle egrets follow the tractors to snatch up the grubs exposed by the plow. Rainfall is timely most of the time in Missouri and irrigation is not often required.

Missouri bottomland and flood plains near the great Missouri and Mississippi Rivers were historically revitalized each year by floods that brought life-giving silt from the Missouri Brakes in Montana (Missouri River) and the Great Lakes north of Ohio (Ohio River to the Mississippi River).

The Missouri summers were hot and humid – the air was hazy and heavy with moisture. I frequently hunted yellow and red winged grasshoppers with a 410-gauge shotgun to hone my dove and quail hunting technique for the coming fall. Tree frogs and cicadas marked their territories with song, screeching and croaking each summer night; fireflies were chased, caught and viewed with wonder in glass jars. Gardens had to be weeded and the first cutting of alfalfa bailed, loaded on the wagons and stored in the barn. You could literally hear the corn squeak as it grew. Bullfrog tadpole's tails were just about absorbed and they would soon be just right for gigging.

The second cutting of hay, the grinding of corn to make silage and fried green tomatoes signaled late summer and the coming of fall. The Missouri fall was bright gold, warm and dry, Indian summer (70 degree weather after a hard frost) was perfect for harvest even until November most years. The hardwood's (oak, hickory, walnut, sweet gum, wild cherry, etc.) leaves turned yellow, orange, red and purple before the leaves browned and fell to the wood's floor and returned minerals and organic matter back to the soil.

The third and sometimes fourth cuttings of alfalfa hay were wind rowed, baled and loaded onto the wagon by hand; corn and soybeans crops harvested each fall were the renewable gold staple that fueled the mid-west livestock industry.

A truck from the Alhoff Brothers Feed store appeared at our place every fall to grind corn, soybeans and alfalfa, add a vitamin/mineral premix and make pellets that were fed to the brood cows and the feeder calves. The vitamin/mineral enriched pellets were a staple for ensuring proper disease free growth for the calves, 100 normal pregnancies from 100 cows, 100 normal calves that were born to 100 cows without the need for a cesarean section and 100 calves that reached market weight or choice heifers that were selected for the breeding herd without the need for veterinary care.

There was a small vein of hard high sulfur coal on our property that was ground into small pea-sized granules and fed free-choice to the cows and calves as another source of minerals – they ate the coal granules with great relish. An analysis showed that coal contained as many as 80 different minerals! Did we need to eat coal?

Rural Missouri winters could be hard, bone chilling cold with deep snow and "black ice" but was often just foggy, wet and drizzly. The woods were naked with all the leaves down with only the occasional squirrel nest and empty bird nests in the branches here and there to give a hint of life. Winter was the time to feed the breeding cows silage that smelled of fermented "corn mash," take every machine and implement apart, change the oil, belts and hoses, cut wood, go to the livestock sale barns to buy or sell cows, bulls and feeder calves and buy seed. We listened to the radio a lot.

The Missouri and Mississippi Rivers, the two dominating, wide, and deep rivers that suckled the soil of the state of Missouri, were tamed by dams and levies in the rivers and creeks bringing water from the water sheds to prevent flooding. The dams also provided a predictable water and electrical supply for the great cities of St. Louis and Kansas City. The river dams controlled the water level of the rivers but in a sinister side effect they also cut off the food supply (mineral rich silt) to downstream bottomland, the Louisiana delta emptying into the Gulf of Mexico and the Atlantic Ocean. We had begun the process of starving ourselves of nutritional minerals!

I was born one and a half years before the attack on Pearl Harbor and I grew up in Missouri raising purebred Angus beef calves and feeder calves in rural west St. Louis County. The feeder calves were fed for six to nine months before they were shipped off to feedlots to be fattened by other feeders or to be butchered. We always saved back the very best ones for our own family. We knocked them in the head and butchered them – a simple cycle on the farm. I learned how to dress and skin a beef carcass and how to inspect the internal organs to assure the animal was disease-free and safe to eat. We sold the skins for cash money.

All four of my grandparents immigrated to St. Louis County from the Ukraine/Romania just before WW I broke out. They were tough yet simple rural people who worked hard. My maternal grandfather and my mother delivered his vegetables and corn to city dwellers with a horse and wagon. He died in his forties from tularemia that he contracted from a minor nick of a jagged bone fragment while skinning a wild rabbit. He probably could have been saved with penicillin. Unfortunately, penicillin hadn't been invented yet. My widowed maternal grandmother survived and raised her three children by gardening, by creating and operating a farmers market and by taking bets on the horse races.

My paternal grandparents raised five kids in a rural-suburban setting. They raised beef, tended a "truck farm" garden and operated a recycling business, known prior to the 60s as the "junk" business. My dad bought and sold calves and "junked" before he got a place of his own. My grandfather died in his eighties from the complications of alcoholism. My paternal grandmother was killed in a nursing home at age 97 from an overdose of insulin administered by one of the nurses.

My dad won the national Golden Gloves boxing championship at the 123-pound weight class in two years in a row at the Madison Square Garden in New York City in 1936 and 1937.

I led a Huckleberry Fynn lifestyle during my early years. We lived in a clapboard house in the hay and cornfields of rural St. Louis County. The hay barn was four times bigger than the house.

We collected rainwater with a roof cistern system that held 500 gallons of water – after five minutes of rain fell to wash the bird droppings off the roof, a valve was turned to collect the water. Our kitchen not only housed the wood stove we used for cooking and heating, it also served as the living room, farm office and laundry room. There was a sagging brass bed at one corner of the kitchen for grandma. We took baths in a galvanized oval washtub in the middle of the kitchen near the warm stove. Water for our baths was heated on the stove. A blue enamel roasting pot was simmering on top of the stove at all times and filled with beef, pork, poultry, herbs and vegetables. Towards the end of each month we were often reduced to eating onion and mustard sandwiches.

We had a wooden icebox that kept our perishable foods cool. The iceman came once each week bringing a load of 50-pound blocks of ice on his red and green horse drawn wagon. On occasion the iceman would bring us gallons of ice cream and stay long enough to have a conversation and bring us news of the outside world. Once he brought a new butter substitute product called margarine. It was soft and lard-like in consistency, white in color and was packaged in a clear soft plastic bag. There was an orange disc the size of a nickel in the bag that contained a yellow food dye – I got to knead the dye throughout the margarine to turn it a butter-like yellow. We never ordered the margarine because my dad said it was only good for caulking the outhouse.

My dad taught me how to work hard, be responsible and how to solve problems small and large – that which was difficult just took a little time; that which was thought by others to be impossible only took a little longer - this "will not be defeated" attitude wasn't empty bravado, it was the way that the west was won!

Although my dad was not a highly educated man in terms of formal schooling he taught me to look forward and to have plan B, C, D, E, F and G in place and ready to put online in case plan A failed to be successful or was insufficient to meet our needs. He didn't depend on others or one source of income for shelter or food for the family – there was farming, livestock, "junking" (called recycling today), contract harvest work for others whose equipment broke down, welding, construction, hauling, he once owned a small restaurant, he was a boxing promoter and manager (Virgil "Honey Bear" Akins, one of his fighters that became the welter weight champion of the world), etc. I acted as a corner man for Sonny Liston when he was only a four round preliminary event fighter.

If there were no sources of money or jobs available locally, my dad would hook his small silver Air Stream trailer to his old rusted out yellow Chevy pickup truck and go to where the work was (lead mining in Kentucky was a common source of cash money for us) and he sent his paycheck home. Once he drove his trailer to the east coast to do welding for submarine construction. We never had a lot of money but we were never really broke and we were always rich in attitude.

My dad's attitude was illustrated by Rudyard Kipling's famous poem "If" – my dad gave me a framed copy of Kipling's poem when I was nine years old and I have carried a small copy with me at all times since and I read it often:

"IF"

If you can keep your head when all about you Are losing theirs and blaming it on you, If you can trust yourself when all men doubt you But make allowance for their doubting too If you can wait and not be tired by waiting, Or being lied about, don't deal in lies, Or being hated, don't give way to hating, And yet don't look too good, nor talk too wise:

If you can dream – and not make dreams your master, If you can think – and not make thoughts your aim;

If you can meet Triumph and Disaster And treat those two imposters just the same;

If you can bear to hear the truth you've spoken Twisted by knaves to make a trap for fools, Or watch the things you gave your life to, broken, And stoop and build 'em up with worn-out tools:

If you can make one heap of all your winnings And risk it all on one turn of pitch-and-toss, And lose, and start again at your beginnings And never breath a word about your loss;

If you can force your heart and nerve and sinew To serve your turn long after they are gone, And so hold on when nothing is in you Except the Will which says to them "Hold on!"

If you can walk with crowds and keep your virtue, Or walk with kings – nor lose the common touch, If neither foes nor loving friends can hurt you;

If all men count with you, but none too much, If you can fill the unforgiving minute With sixty seconds' worth of distance run, Yours is the Earth and everything that's in it, And – which is more – you'll be a Man, my son!

My grandmothers were my early playmates – we played hide and seek, worked jigsaw puzzles, played cards, checkers, chess, assembled erector sets, played pick-up sticks and read books to each other. They started me on my chores feeding the chickens, milking cows and feeding calves. They taught me how to fire up the wood stove, snap beans, shuck corn, cook, can and store food, make lye soap using wood ash, do laundry, weed the garden and gather berries, mushrooms, wild onions and herbs. Their kitchens were comfortable and smelled of orange skins and cloves that were heated on the top of the wood stove and of baking bread and cookies.

I was charged with keeping the kitchen wood box and coal bin full. I collected wood scraps from the sawmill down the road and gathered branches from the nearby woods and cut them to the proper length with an axe; larger pieces of firewood were split with steel wedges and a hammer. I kept a chunk of the calves trace mineral salt block in my overall pocket and sucked on it while I worked; in the summer when I could get it I chewed melted road tar – I learned later that these cravings for salt, minerals and tar were caused by mineral deficiencies and known in animals as cribbing or pica.

I was also responsible for cleaning the wood stove each day and putting the previous days wood ashes in the garden. Wood ashes were fine powdered minerals that were left in the stove after the fire burned off the woody carbon - we used the ashes along with compost and manure to fertilize the garden.

Even at the age of six I contributed to the welfare of the family by bringing home fish (catfish, bluegill, sunfish, crappie, small mouth bass, perch), eels, turtles, crawdads and bullfrogs. At age ten I was an accomplished marksman and hunter and brought home rabbits, squirrels, raccoon, possum, doves, pigeons and quail. I trapped muskrats and sold the skins. At age 14 I killed my first deer.

I built a 6 foot by 10 foot raft of empty five-gallon farm chemical cans held together in a frame and covered with raw planks – when not doing my chores I was a river rat. I built a shelter on the raft and on weekends stayed overnight on the water when I could – I became self reliant and unafraid to take to the sloughs and rivers by myself.

By 12 years of age I could rope and drop a running 600-pound steer in his tracks. I learned how to halter break calves, groom them, trim their feet, dehorn them when necessary and prepare them for show and sale.

I joined the boy scouts with Troop 495 sponsored by the Blackberry Lane elementary School in St. Louis County. Our scout master was Sydney Jacobs, a former marine captain from World War II – our 300 strong scout troop became what I can only describe as a crack paramilitary unit complete with a drum and bugle corps. We always wore complete class-A uniforms with spit-shined brown leather shoes and polished brass – there were no blue jeans or tennis shoes in Troop 495.

We could compete with any professional drill team. We attended weeklong summer camps often times doing two weeks back to back, weekend camping events and took 30-mile marches with full field packs for fun, but we also developed our tracking, observational and survival skills. We developed individual pride and confidence, team pride and confidence and a "can do," leave no man behind and will not be defeated spirit.

I became an Eagle Scout after being forced by my dad and Sydney Jacobs to overcome my inability to swim and master the required swimming and lifesaving merit badges; I collected, catalogued and mounted insects, butterflies, leaves, feathers, fossils, rocks, mineral ores and bones. These organizational, cataloging, detail and observational habits and skills eventually led to the EPIPHANY, which began as the simple observations of a teenager feeding mineral supplements to beef calves.

We went to great pains to get supplemental minerals into our cattle but did not give ourselves the same supplementation, yet we ate corn and garden vegetables from the same fields. Why did the calves require supplemental minerals and we didn't?

As a teen-ager I suffered from eyelid twitches that were so severe you could hear them click. The eye doctor felt the twitches were due to my eyelashes hitting my glasses and curling back and tickling my eye – she actually wanted me to use a mascara brush to retrain my eyelashes. I went to the high school library and looked up muscle twitches and cramps and learned that they were caused by a simple calcium deficiency.

I went straight home from the library to the barn and filled my pockets with calcium enriched calf pellets and ate them through the day like candy – the twitches went away.

The grade school, high school, university and scientific communities' mantra has been historically and is yet today "we can get everything we need from our basic four food groups." However, if one looks at the score card, we immediately see that the concept that one "can get everything they need from the basic four food groups" has killed more Americans than all of the wars, terrorist acts and muggings that have occurred in the 220 years since we became a nation!

Although Americans have had the most food and the highest quality food than any other country over the 220 years we have been a nation, we still only average 75.5 years of age (half of our genetic potential for 120 – 140 years) and rank only 24th in the world for longevity – there are 23 other countries whose peoples live longer than we do!

Throw in the most expensive and the most technologically advanced health care system in the world we still make no gains when it comes to health and longevity because doctors kill between 150,000 and 300,000 Americans each year in hospitals alone.

Before graduating high school my first paying job off the farm was a job at the St. Louis Zoo – I was hired over thousands of other applicants because I had experience working with large animals and was "willing to do anything necessary" to work with Marlin Perkins, director of the St. Louis Zoo and host of Mutual of Omaha's Wild Kingdom.

My first task was to bottle-raise two baby Asian elephants (Florence and Pearl) under the watchful eye of the legendary elephant trainer Floyd Smith. Floyd was the only individual to successfully hand raise baby elephants to adulthood. His secret was "blue" clay – yep, he insisted that the baby elephants would not survive without their daily ration of "blue" clay.

I dug a bucketful of "blue" clay every week from a far corner of the zoo and dutifully fed an orange-sized ball to each baby every day – which by the way they eagerly ate like candy. I learned several years later that "blue" clay contains a wide variety of major and trace minerals! Did humans need "blue" clay? I took little pea-sized nibbles of the clay into my mouth each day and swallowed them.

When I reached the age of 16 I was allowed to work with the

seven adult Asian show elephants. Have you ever wondered why elephants don't drop manure on the stage while they are performing – it's because there is a 16 year old behind the scenes manually removing the manure from their rectums! Three times each day, Monday through Saturday and four times on Sunday the job was done without fail June through September.

In high school I wrestled at 123 pounds for the Clayton Greyhounds and became captain of the wrestling team. I played offensive center and left guard and middle line backer on the defensive squad in football and lettered in football at only 123 pounds; and I weight lifted and became familiar with various brands of food supplements used by athletes. Body builders seemed more interested in vitamin-mineral supplements than athletes in other sports who were more interested in "strength training."

My dad had started me on vitamin-mineral supplements when I was only six and I took them because he was bigger than me; but I really started taking supplements in earnest in high school – I played hard yet never suffered the injuries that plagued the larger and more talented athletes. I was physically durable because I trained hard and supplemented with vitamins and minerals with intensity.

After graduating high school in 1958 I went on to enroll in the school of agriculture at the University of Missouri where I studied animal husbandry, nutrition, soils, soil chemistry and how to maximize yields in terms of tons and bushels per acre. We learned how to maximize fertility in herd bulls, rams and boars and brood cows, ewes, mares and sows and how to improve general herd health, genetics (selective breeding), increase muscle mass, increase the immune status, eliminate degenerative diseases in livestock and save the farmer money at the same time.

I subsidized my schooling by working for the dairy department and the beef departments doing feed studies, production performance studies and daily chores. These jobs were comfortable because it was what I had done at home.

Dr. William Albrecht, my soils professor, made it clear that all soils were not equal and that the food value of wheat or beans grown in one field were not necessarily the same as the food value of wheat or beans grown in another field. It became obvious to me that every animal and every human needed to supplement with vitamins and minerals – food alone couldn't meet our daily needs!

Albrecht pointed out that cattle and sheep tended to eat and graze from particular areas of a pasture that were rich in minerals and shunned parts of the pastures that were mineral deficient and that we were obligated to make up the deference in mineral values of livestock feed by supplementing the soil and the feed to have uniform health and production in livestock. Albrecht's observations began to explain why we gave minerals to our calves – but why didn't we take minerals ourselves?

I learned in essence that the health and longevity in all species depends on the mineral content of thin crust on the earth's surface. To maximize the earth's yields in terms of tons, bushels, dozens, gallons and pounds we learned that we had to supplement the soil and animal feed with nutrients that were found in either low concentrations or were totally missing from the soil. The EPIPHANY was now taking real form and was being supported by an accumulation of real data and numbers.

Chapter 10

Ten Rhino at Palumbo

"The beauty and genius of a work of art may be reconceived though its first material expression be destroyed; a vanished harmony may yet again inspire the composer; but when the last individual of a race of living things breathes no more, another heaven and another earth must pass before such a one can be again."

—William Beebe
Bronx Zoo

In veterinary school at the University of Missouri we learned that we could economically add healthful productive years to the longevity of a breeding herd of livestock, laboratory and pet animals simply by eliminating disease – and we did it by the use of simple nutritional formulas – mouse pellets, rat pellets, hamster pellets, guinea pig pellets, rabbit pellets, canned and dry dog and cat food, calf pellets, sheep pellets, pig pellets, horse pellets, pigeon pellets, turkey pellets, chicken pellets, duck pellets, monkey pellets, catfish pellets, etc.

The use of complete feed pellets guaranteed that each animal, even the most silly or stupid one in each group, flock or herd, the most dominant or the most dominated would get a perfect diet in each mouthful. Pellets prevented the animals from sorting through feed and eating only the corn, sunflower seeds or soybeans; pellets prevented the avoidance of vitamin and mineral supplements – each animal is forced to eat a perfect diet! Farmers did not let their incomes or financial survival depend on the whims or choices of the animals themselves!

A 10-year old dog was an old dog in the 1930s, today an old dog is 20 years old; a 10-year old cat was an old cat in the 1930s, today an old cat is 26 years old. Extended longevity in animals was brought about with simple yet complete nutritional supplements, not genetic engineering. Dogs and cats had always possessed the genetic potential to live beyond 20 years of age but it took serious nutritional science to allow them to fulfill their genetic potential for longevity! No raw materials – no product!

If we could so easily eliminate disease and early death in animals with simple nutritional formulas, why didn't we do the same for human populations? The question came up again and again, "Why didn't medical doctors talk about vitamins and minerals?"

In addition to my veterinary studies I pursued graduate pathology courses after graduating from agriculture school in 1962, studying animal and human disease. It soon became clear through animal and human autopsies that nutritional deficiency diseases were a serious health and economic threat to animal and human populations.

My mentor and instructor in veterinary pathology was Dr. Loren Kintner. Dr. Kintner took me on as a student assistant when I showed an aptitude for following clues to an end point, seeing minute gross and microscopic tissue changes, recording details and a zeal for studying pathology.

Beginning in the summer of my sophomore year in vet school (after I had graduated agriculture school in 1962), under the supervision of Dr. Kintner, I did the gross and microscopic pathology for the veterinary school small and large animal clinics, veterinary and medical research projects, wildlife (deer, coyote, fox, bobcat, raccoon, possum, beaver, owls, hawks, ducks, geese, wild turkey, fish, snakes, turtles, frogs, salamanders) from the school of forestry and service pathology for farmers and veterinarians around the state of Missouri.

Dr. Kintner taught me to be a relentless and uncompromising detective, to look for the truth rather than accept common belief and theory, to examine every detail before drawing a conclusion

– Sherlock Holmes became my literary hero. "Eliminate the impossible and what ever is left, no matter how improbable must be the truth!" said Holmes.

Sometimes I performed as many as 25 autopsies per day. Farmers could bring in a pickup truck full of dead pigs, lambs or turkeys. Each carcass was carefully given a full autopsy; cultures were taken from the intestines, blood, organs and lesions to search for microorganisms, tissue samples were taken for microscopic and toxicology examination. The sheer volume of the autopsies gave me an understanding, experience and skill that few could ever hope to have. Most medical students memorize the names of disease - I understood disease!

After graduating veterinary school, with the help of Dr. Kintner, I took a job in Ames, Iowa and taught pathology to graduate students and senior veterinary students at the veterinary school at Iowa State University and performed service pathology at the Iowa State Diagnostic Laboratory for the regional farm community, veterinarians, the university wildlife department and medical research projects.

While teaching pathology at Iowa State I continued my graduate work by taking comparative anatomy and pathology courses under the tutorage of two nationally known and respected pathologists Dr. Frank Ramsey and Dr. Vaughn Seaton – deepening my interest and understanding of diseases in animals and people that were caused by nutritional deficiencies.

The other pathology grad students in the "stable" were more interested in the academics of pathology than in the blood and guts of pathology – they wanted to be teachers; I just wanted to fully understand disease. As a result of their disinterest in doing autopsies they often asked me to take on all of their autopsy cases – I performed as many as 10 to 25 autopsy cases each day; some cases consisted of one cow, some cases consisted of a pickup truck full of baby pigs or lambs.

After one year at The Iowa State University Diagnostic Laboratory I had the opportunity to go to South Africa and work on conservation projects for the white rhino and elephant. With the help of my mentor, Marlin Perkins – the director of the St. Louis Zoological Gardens and the famed host of the TV series Wild Kingdom, my farm background and my wildlife pathology skills, I got the job.

After a short three-month stint as a government veterinarian monitoring foot and mouth disease in domestic animals and wildlife in South Africa, I was transferred to the service of the Natal Parks Board as the veterinarian for Operation Rhino. The white rhino was crowded out of its original home range by crops and orchards. Twentieth century poachers armed with modern firearms hunted the rhino for his horn without concern for the long – term survival of the species.

By 1896 the white rhino was officially thought to be extinct until a small herd was located in a minute triangle of land framed by the White and Black Umfolozi Rivers in Zululand near the east coast of Natal Province, the lush mid-eastern province of the Republic of South Africa.

An official count of the white rhino population uncovered only 20 individual rhino in the area near the junction of the two rivers. This unexpected discovery in 1897 led to the establishment of crown land to protect the species from final extinction. The charter of the Umfolozi and Hluhluwe game parks soon followed to allow public viewing of the great beasts.

Operation Rhino was a bold project devoted to saving the white rhino from extinction. Totally dependent on their nutritional survival by the grazing of one species of short grass, the fragile white rhino population was at risk of final doom from the competitive grazing of wart hogs, antelope, Cape buffalo, domestic cattle and goats and slash and burn farming.

Operation Rhino consisted of two parts: 1) Eliminate the rhino's competitors and enhance the rhino's home range; 2) Establish breeding herds of the white rhino in many locations so that "all the eggs weren't in one basket." The elimination of the white rhino's competitors and enhancing their home range was easy and the system was already proven in other species. The establishment of breeding herds of the rare white rhino in numerous locations was impossible until the advent of the tranquilizer gun and the discovery of a potent tranquilizer that could immobilize the large rhino with small doses that would fit in the tiny darts.

I officially became a game ranger in the Natal Game and Fish Department. My job responsibilities were to first and foremost save the white rhino from extinction, provide veterinary care for the game park's 200 head of horses, mules and donkeys and as a science officer collect blood samples, ticks, water samples and foliage samples to monitor disease and gauge the ability of the park to support rhino.

Ranger John Clark was the rhino expert in the Umfolozi and Hluhluwe Game Reserves and I became his student. I already knew the basics of firearms and tracking from my hunting experience in Missouri and from my boy scout training; I was a very good shot and not afraid of large animals because of my experience with cattle and zoo elephants – I just had to learn how the immobilizing drugs worked and the way rhino thought and their physical abilities and limits.

Before I even unpacked my gear we were off catching rhino and I became a student again. After a week of watching and learning I began to catch rhino on my own. After a month on the job, John got married and ran off on his honeymoon for 30 days and I became a rhino catching expert.

When John returned from his honeymoon, we had one of the greatest adventures recorded in the history of animal conservation – Ten Rhino at Palumbo! The adventure was initiated by the white rhino's seasonal migration to the south. The annual migration was anticipated with some aversion by the Umfolozi rangers. These annual marches left ruptured border fences and sparked some rather colorful complaints from the Zulu subsistence farmers in the Palumbo Native Location. On the map the Umfolozi Game Reserve and the Palumbo Native Locations were very distinct and separate pieces of real estate. In reality, on the ground, the two different spots on the map were only separated and divided by a four-strand 5/8-inch steel cable fence.

The cable fence was erected in hopes of discouraging the rhino from gravitating south back into the native reserve. To date, the fence has only acted effectively as a boundary marker. The rhino's determination to reach the low veldt at Palumbo was so determined that it took the animal only a few days work to lift the fence poles out of the ground. As if drawn by some beacon known only to them, large numbers of rhino would find the break and pour through.

Constant fence patrols by the game scouts of the Ogome Ranger Station were necessary to guarantee the integrity of this cable barrier. Large depots of fence posts and cable were stored at strategic points where rhino had broken through in the past.

Once an uprooted pole or broken cable was reported, it was up to the station ranger to get his fence crew organized and repair the damage. When not repairing fence line, these crews were kept busy clearing brush to enable dormant grass seeds laying in the shaded soil to germinate or building stone weirs in heavily eroded areas to collect silt during the rainy season and rebuild soil.

The daily duties of Operation Rhino, while normally a steady routine, often times provided adventures that many young men dream of, but few are ever able to participate in. One such adventure was the record setting rhino catching expedition that became a legend – "Ten Rhino at Palumbo!"

At the request of the Palumbo district headman, the Umfolozi game ranger John Clark and I organized a three-day rhino catch to remove many Mkhombe (Zulu for white rhino) from the kraal's mealie (corn) fields.

Apparently several white rhino had decided to use the fields as a shortcut to reach water from their favorite grazing and resting sites. The rhino also ate the sprouting mealies and damaged the mature stalks in their treks back and forth, and their presence kept the village's women from working in the fields.

When possible we preferred to put rhino that were caught outside the reserve's fence into bomas or pens for training prior to ocean shipping or directly on a truck bound for another nearby reserve. Tagging studies had shown that a considerable percentage of the animals that were returned to Umfolozi had wandered out again. It was unfortunate that our Umfolozi bomas were full and therefore we had no alternative but to release the rhino we caught back into the reserve.

We left Umfolozi before dawn and arrived at the Ogome Ranger Station at about 10:00 a.m. and had tea while the game scouts unloaded our gear. The station consisted of a five-room house, an office, a radio shack and a series of sheds that were used for the station's horses and their tack. The resident ranger was on leave, however, his houseboy extended his bosses' hospitality and took our duffels inside and set up our cots on the screened in veranda.

Moses, our driver, and the heavy Bedford lorry eventually arrived with an empty rhino crate and a complement of six boma laborers. We climbed into the vehicle and headed south, through the southern most extension of the Umfolozi Reserve. The route to the Palumbo district was a rugged boulder-strewn area with heavy brush that provided a perfect habitat for nyala, greater kudu, bushbuck and waterbuck.

We arrived at the Palumbo district kraal at about noon to start the rhino rescue operation; as we got out of the truck, our crew was immediately surrounded by a crowd of villagers. The headman stoically stepped forward and identified himself - he wore the impeccable uniform of a British First World War cavalry officer. He introduced himself in French and when we acknowledged his lingual superiority, he smiled and proceeded to try me at German, Portuguese and Afrikaans, before resorting to English with a disappointed sigh.

He told us of at least eight white rhino that were trampling the kraal's mealies in their daily excursions. While he talked, I made up two tranquilizer darts and filled each of them with enough drugs to immobilize adult rhino. Once our preparations were completed and the catching equipment checked, we followed the scouts out of the village and across several freshly plowed fields.

We were led to a small patch of veldt between two sprouted mealie fields, where two small herds of rhino were having a late morning siesta. They were resting on the bare earth created by the shade of a lone acacia tree. The dusty, well, worn loafing area was surrounded by grass and a slight wind was angling from us to the sleeping rhino. John and I circled to get downwind and stalked to within 20 yards of the larger group.

The rhino were grunting and blowing in a relaxed fashion, totally unaware of our presence and intent. We sat for a moment to catch our breath and survey the situation. This group consisted of four animals, a large bull lying broadside to the left and three animals sleeping in a line shoulder to shoulder facing us just off to the right by about 10 yards.

By finger drawings in the dust, we agreed that John would dart the bull on the left and I would take the largest of the three rhino on the right. I counted to three in a whisper, and we fired our darts simultaneously – John's dart struck the bull in the left shoulder and my dart hit its mark in the junction of the neck and shoulder of the second animal.

The startled rhino jumped to their feet with a snort and a cloud of dust and headed off into the wind immediately. Our mounted game scouts followed at a gallop close behind, but John and I were momentarily cut off from following by the second upper herd as they cut back diagonally down the hill with the wind.

We skirted the approaching rhino and came up on the original group at a tree line. We found the two darted rhino lying down less than 30 yards apart in a small clearing. We chased off the two smaller rhino and instructed the horsemen to keep tabs on them for later attention. John ran off to find Moses and the lorry while the headman and I talked about rhino.

We loaded and sent off the first rhino and it was well after 1:00 p.m. when the lorry returned to pick up the second rhino for release into the Umfolozi Reserve. While the rhino was being loaded, I made up two more darts and then followed the horse's tracks into a wide thicket of low acacia bush. By now the heat of the day was at its peak, and a shattering beat was coming from the "Christmas bees."

The insects were not actually bees, but summer cicadas. Each summer the male insects produce a tireless screech, not unlike a sound made by a worn out water pump on a car. The purpose of the call was to attract receptive females. Combined with the heat waves rising off the bush veldt, the noise gave an eerie background to stalking rhino through the dense brush on hands and knees.

After an hour's tracking, we spotted four animals 15 yards ahead resting in the sparse shade afforded by several twisted acacia. In whispers, we made our plans. I was to remain behind while John circled to the right and downwind of the herd. After he signaled that he was in position I was to dart an animal and he would dart another as the herd passed him downwind in their attempt to escape.

At John's whistle, the quizzical rhino stood up and moved a few steps into the bush. The cheek of a large cow presented me with my only clear shot. I could barely make out the outline of her large gray head through a small 10-inch opening in the bush. I aimed the dart at her taut check and pulled the trigger – the dart hit with a loud schluup, and I feared at first that the dart had hit her ear and the drug had been ejected harmlessly into the external ear canal.

The darted cow reversed her direction and led the other rhino in the opposite direction from John, who stood up and took a chance shot that hit a tree limb.

The darted cow went down peacefully on the edge of a donga (dry arroyo) in about 10 minutes. Her 900-pound calf stayed close by, so I quickly prepared a dart for it and another for an adult animal. While I worked, two bulls noiselessly made their way toward the donga.

John darted the calf and I darted one of the two half-grown bulls that had stepped out of the bush in response to the calf's frantic calls. The bull, stung by the dart, brushed the irritating object out of his hide as he made his way back through the bush. When I picked up the dart and examined it, I found that the percussion cap had failed to go off. In the meantime, the calf had followed the two bulls back into the open veldt, where it went down hard on its side, throwing up a cloud of dust. The two curious bulls turned back and hung around to see why the calf had gone to sleep so early and so suddenly.

I rammed the misfired dart back into the gun and stepped out from the cover of the bush and darted the nearest bull as he started to trot off. At the missile's impact, the astounded rhino stopped, whirled around to face me and stared. After a 10-minute wait, it was apparent that the percussion cap was faulty and it hadn't gone off for the second time.

I moved around downwind and went to the Land Rover that Moses had thoughtfully brought up and quickly prepared another dart. On returning, the rhino caught my scent and turned defiantly in my direction. This again necessitated approaching in a wide semicircle before I could come into range without scaring the two bulls off. I crawled back into the cover of the bush where John was waiting and loaded the capture gun.

I moved forward on my hands and knees through the thick underbrush so I could get a clear shot at the bulls shoulder. At a distance of 16 yards, all I could see of the six-foot animal was his feet. When I rose up on one knee to shoot, the bulls turned and ran toward me! I fired the dart into the lead rhino's shoulder; the dart hung there just momentarily before being flipped out by the violent movements of the bull's charge. The old question of, "did the animal get the full dose of the drug or not?" came up again, and this was no doubt our last crack at him that day as it was getting windy and very rapidly turning dark.

John and I waited under the bush for a long five minutes. Still the darted rhino stood and stared in our direction. Then he awkwardly took two goose-steps forward, and we sighed in relief – he was showing the signs of being drugged. He walked towards our bush in exaggerated steps, passing within a few yards of us while his companion galloped in wide circles, bellowing and tossing his head. We reluctantly watched the horsemen chase him off, but as it was, we would do well to get three sleeping rhino out of the bush that night using only the lights of the Land Rover without a mishap.

When our lone lorry returned and Moses saw the three rhino down, he shook his head and volunteered a pessimistic, "Whoa, whoa – this is the day we die," meaning that John and I were going to work him and his crew to death. We loaded the bull first and put an anchor rope on the cow and calf. John took a turn at guard duty while I went with Moses and the lorry to supervise the bull's release on a dry riverbank so we would not have to waste precious time completely off-loading and reloading the crate.

When Moses and I returned to the downed rhino, it was pitch dark. Since we had been without food and water for nearly 14 hours, John, to kill time, had been exploring the streambed for water. I found him on his knees digging in some likely looking wet sand. At a depth of one foot, cool black water began slowly filling the cone-shaped hole.

The water was cool and slightly salty, but it was a very refreshing treat even though we were only able to get a few ounces each.

John took the cow for release while I stayed back with the calf. When John, Moses and the lorry returned at 8:30 p.m., the bull's companion had appeared again looking for his chum, and the calf was beginning to come around and cry out in a plaintive call for help.

We had to sit on the calf to keep her down while the crate was unloaded. She was hustled quickly into the oversized crate, the procedure being aided by her alert state. Soon we were heading back with our small caravan of lorry, Rover and horsemen, all tired but jubilant because we had set a record of five rhino caught and moved in one day – and with only one lorry (I am sure our record still stands today).

We arrived at the Ogome Ranger Station at 10:00 p.m. We took turns having a muddy but welcome bath; we raided the station's icebox, then we unceremoniously flopped into our cots where sleep came quickly.

We were awakened at sunrise by the braying arrival of the mule drawn water wagon coming up the hill from the White Umfolozi River. Each morning 300 gallons of the brown river water were collected and hauled to the top of the hill to supply the daily needs of the outpost. In addition to meeting the needs of the residents of the station, the horses, donkeys, mules and flowers all required their daily ration of water.

While enjoying the pleasant jingling of the mule harness, I shaved, I dressed and then cleaned the used darts and put them to boiling while we ate a hearty breakfast of warthog, eggs and potatoes.

Once again we headed south for the Palumbo kraals. On arriving at the store, our scouts informed us that a small group of three rhino were resting up in a dense patch of bush only a quarter of a mile away. The headman waved his arms about while relating the great deeds of yesterday to a growing and eager audience. I assembled two darts with green flights for adult rhino and two with white flights for yearlings, since the trackers' descriptions did not include the rhino's size or age.

We walked in single file down a dusty village path. At a nod from the head tracker, we crept into the tangle of acacia thorn with dry twigs and fallen leaves crackling loudly underfoot. As the sun rose higher, the "Christmas bees" added their shrieking to our noise. The combination of the throbbing background noise and the distortion of the heat waves in the air began playing tricks on our now tired nerves – and we came around the screen of each bush expecting a rhino.

Finally, we found the three rhino dozing – a large bull standing and a cow and calf lying down. The three animals were ahead and to our left, and so far were unaware that they had been discovered. John was in a good position to dart the bull, so without hesitation he took his shot. The unexpected slap of the dart surprised the bull and caused him to back into the cow. She stood up with a start, agitated at the bull's apparent clumsiness and bad manners. John then darted the cow in the shoulder with the calf dose in hopes of slowing her down. As soon as I saw his dart hit the cow, I stepped forward and tried to dart her with the second calf dart, but it hit at a bad angle and glanced off her rump and just added speed to her exit!

We cast about, looking for the bull's tracks for a few moments, but gave up in the maze of gravel and dry leaves. We returned to the vehicles, where I made up another dart for a calf. I gave John the adult dart that I had previously made and loaded up with the calf load and we set off into the bush. After walking a mile north, one of our horsemen clattered up loudly, telling us that the bull was down. We told him to go back and guard it lest local horn hunters took the opportunity to chop up the unprotected rhino with cane knives in its drugged state.

The second horseman appeared just as the first rider left and breathlessly told us that the cow had stopped against a tree about two miles away. When we arrived, we found the cow down on her brisket but not completely out; we attached an anchor rope to her rear leg and tied her to a nearby tree. It was a simple matter to dart the calf as it stayed defiantly near its mother.

By chance, a lone bull emerged from the bush, which John handily darted. By one o'clock in the afternoon we had four animals down.

Extracting the four rhino proved to be difficult as the lorry crew had to hack roads through the tangled thorn so the lorry could be backed up right to the bull that John had originally darted. After administering the antidote it took an unusually long hour to get him loaded into the crate and the crate back up on the truck. While the lorry went off to drop the first rhino inside the Umfolozi fence, the cow stood up, swaying at the end of her tether, so I gave her an additional dose of drug with a hand syringe. The horsemen had lazily watched the cow go down again and had momentarily taken their eyes off of the calf. As I pulled the original dart from the calf's skin it jumped up and caught the distracted men flat-footed, the horses alert, though, pulled the men out of the calf's way just in time. I gave the calf an additional dose to get it under control.

The lorry returned and we loaded the cow into crate and levered the sweating calf onto the bed of the Land Rover, where it was lashed down with heavy rope. We offloaded the cow and calf in Umfolozi and headed back for Palumbo.

When we returned for the bull, we found it impossible to locate any suitable place for a road to be cut because of a heavy rock outcropping and several large trees. We voted unanimously for walking the bull down a dry riverbed that was handy, a half-mile from the nearest road where we could have the crate ready.

While Moses left with the lorry to get the crate in position on the road, John and I took a 30-foot 3/8 inch hemp rope and a 50 foot ½ inch nylon rope and headed back toward the rhino. We put a slipknot in the nylon rope and placed it over the bull's head just behind his posterior horn. The hemp rope we tied around his left rear leg as a drag- line.

We were able to bring the blinking animal to its feet without any antidote – he had been down for five hours and the affects of the drugs were wearing off. With hearty shouts and vigorous slaps behind the ears, we drove him the 15 yards to the riverbed. We had to use long tree limbs to leverage him down the three-foot embankment into the dry river. He crumpled into the dry river sand in a heap and a cloud of dust and sand. After recovering his feet, he initially headed in the wrong direction so we had to redirect him by pulling on his tail and the leg rope.

With six men pulling in front and three behind acting as anchor men or prodders as the situation required, we moved the bull down the dry river the one half mile to the road in an hour. The roughest part was yet to come – the mature 5,000 - pound bull was now regaining his faculties and more actively resisting our guidance, and we had yet to get him back up the riverbank and into the narrow opening of the crate.

We hauled the lead rope through the crate and out the hole in the front door and anchored it to the rear axel of the lorry. On signal, we prodded and worried the bull with words until he lumbered up the bank under his own power and into the sanctuary of the crate to escape his tormentors.

Before we could react quickly enough to latch the rear door behind him, and before the lorry was able to move forward and collect the slack in the rope, the bull rebounded off the front door and backed up, snapping the half inch nylon rope like it was fishing line. He quickly retreated, pulling the six straining Zulu laborers holding the rope up against the front of the crate like so many seeds pealed off along a grass stem. After a brief moment of chaos and pandemonium, we finally collected ourselves and pushed the bellowing animal back into the crate.

After two hard, record-breaking days, the lorry crew was now thoroughly exhausted. They fell silent, so I had Moses promise them soft drinks and strike up a sing-song chant. John and I pitched in and picked up the heavy ends of the steel loading rollers, which no doubt helped to boost their flagging spirits.

We happily let the bull loose in Umfolozi and returned to the Ogome Ranger Station just after full darkness. We traded stories and had a glorious dinner of stuffed wildebeest heart, mealie porridge and beer. On a comfortably full stomach I crawled into bed and oblivion.

The third morning it took several hours to clean up, clean the dirty dart guns and gather up the tired laborers so we only arrived at the Palumbo store after 11:30 a.m.

The headman was patiently waiting for us as usual on the veranda of the store in his uniform. He said that his trackers had spotted three rhino lying up where we had darted our first rhino two days earlier. After one hour of unproductive creeping about in the bush with the infernal "Christmas bees" screeching in our ears, we learned from one game scout that the local teenagers had thought that rhino catching looked like such good sport that they had tried their skills and had chased the rhino all morning with their dogs.

Frustrated, we climbed into our vehicles and started to drive to the opposite end of the Palumbo location, hoping to head off the rhino's retreat. After a short drive we came upon a lone bull standing in the shade of a small thorn bush just off the track about three hundred yards ahead. We stopped the Rover and signaled for Moses to shut off the lorry. John and I loaded our capture guns and stalked to within 25 yards of the bull before he sensed our presence.

There was a large clump of scrub between the bull and us. We flipped a coin and decided that if the bull chose to go to the right I would take the shot; if he went to the left, John would take it. After a two-minute appraisal of us, the bull curled his tail over his back and trotted off to the right. I let go my dart hitting him just behind the shoulder.

The bull continued on his way at a rapid pace. It was obvious we wouldn't be able to keep up with him on foot, so we waited for the appearance of our vehicles while the horsemen did their job. After an hour, the first horseman returned on his sweating mount, saying that he had found the bull grazing in a clearing, but that the dart had fallen out and the bull was showing no signs of being drugged.

We were discouraged and I was about to set up again when the second horseman came up at a hard gallop, saying he had the rhino sighted about four miles away with the dart still in it. The first rider had apparently stumbled onto yet another animal. The horseman related to us that the bull was still standing and when he had dismounted and tried to put an anchor rope around a rear leg, it had given him a halfhearted charge.

We jumped into our vehicles and, since we now knew the rhino's location, we took a short cut. We found that the bull had made two right angle turns when he had successfully lost one rider earlier in the day.

After arriving at the appointed location, there was some loud confusion about which thicket the bull had been sighted in. We finally had to resort to backtracking the horse in order to find the rhino. We came upon the bull lying down in a patch of sparse bush. He did not look like a typically drugged animal, since he was alertly moving his ears to chase flies off and catch danger signals.

After I loaded another dart, we approached the bull. When we got within arms reach I slapped the rhino on the rump. The response was immediate and loud. The startled rhino, the original dart still in his shoulder, clambered to his feet, bellowing; for a moment he was confused as to which way to run, turning first left, then right. I held off darting him, since at that short range the dart would have exploded on impact and the rhino would surely recognize the direction from were it had come and counter attack!

As the rhino bolted off, he bowled over a dead tree, reducing it to a heap of dust and splinters. As he reached the other side of the clearing, I aimed for the center of his disappearing rump so I would hit him if he zigged or zagged.

The bull chose to go straight so the dart struck him directly in the base of the tail. The animal stopped in the far thicket and turned to look back into the clearing. In about five minutes, he started goose-stepping and wandered back into the open. We simply had to lean against a tree and wait for him to go down. After he crossed the clearing, we realized it would be faster loading if he were headed into the clearing instead of the bush, so with a bit of tail pulling, and grunting, we were able to turn him just as he crashed heavily to the ground.

I pulled out the original dart for examination to find that it had a faulty detonator in it that had failed to go off! The horseman had tried to put a rope around the leg of an un-drugged, exhausted and indignantly surprised rhino, and it was considered fortunate for the rider to leave unscathed. We stalked an un-drugged rhino, "counted coup" on him to use the American Indian term and had escaped the rhino's wrath for reasons only he knew. This last bull was the tenth rhino at Palumbo – the legend is now part of African conservation history.

In addition to the catching, marking, tracking and trans-locating rhino, elephant and antelope, the African conservation project allowed me to continue performing autopsies in large numbers of free ranging animals of many species.

At night we would kill as many as 300 impala and dozens of wildebeest and zebra to manage the herd sizes (each one would be autopsied, blood samples, parasites and ticks were collected to monitor hoof and mouth and other diseases); additionally we killed and ate warthogs to reduce the browsing and grazing pressure on the parched South African veldt and savannah and to reduce space and feed competitors of the white rhino. Our focus was to save the rare and endangered white rhino and it's habitat at all cost.

Plant biomass in the parks would be totally devastated and cropped to the ground by overpopulations of impala, wildebeest, zebra and warthogs leaving only parched dessert sand with no organic material to hold water and give life to the sand. It would take a thousand years, maybe never, to restore the soil and re-grow a dry devastated savannah brush habitat – it only took 20 years to rebuild an animal population so our choices were quite clear.

Each animal killed was autopsied and examined for infectious disease, intestinal and blood parasites, ticks, degenerative diseases, nutritional diseases and general state of health. The meat was cut into strips and dried into jerky-like "biltong"; trophy horns, warthog tusks and all skins were tanned and sold to finance the rhino conservation projects.

Wild animals drank preferentially from rivers, pans or waterholes that were muddy and heavy with mineral silt; the grasses and brush around the silt and mud choked rivers and pans were "hammered" or eaten down to the bare ground, while grass and brush around clear soft water rivers and pans grew "as high as an elephants eye" and were completely ignored by even the hungriest of animals.

Termite nests were a universal attraction for all species of mammals and birds. The two to six foot tall pyramid shaped termite nests were the "tailings" resulting from the termites tunnel excavations. The termite mounds were collections of clay and pulverized rock dust chewed and ground to talcum-sized particles and bonded together by termite saliva.

Elephant, rhino, giraffe, the larger antelope, ostrich, parrots and storks would knock the termite mounds over, crush them with their feet, horns, tusks and beaks and eat the small chunks. Antelope, zebra, monkeys, smaller animals and birds would follow the larger animals and eat the smallest pieces of the pulverized termite nests. This termite nest eating seemed to me to be the equivalent of the St. Louis Zoo's elephant trainer Floyd Smith's "blue clay" supplement program required for raising baby elephants!

What I learned was that free ranging animals living in supposed idyllic circumstances in their natural habitat still exhibited pica and cribbing behavior, still sought out mineral sources and still suffered from mineral nutritional deficiency diseases just like domestic livestock, lab animals, zoo animals, pets and yes humans – the EPIPHANY was universal!

Chapter 11

The Hunt

"Is it really so stupid to work for the zebras, lions, and men who will walk the earth fifty years from now, and for a hundred or two hundred years time?"

—Bernard Grzimek
Frankfort Zoo

Because of my success in the white and black rhino conservation projects in Umfolozi and Hluhluwe Game Reserves in Natal I was invited to participate in a fledgling elephant tagging, cold branding and migration project in the Wankie Game Reserve of Southern Rhodesia (today called Zimbabwe).

Immobilizing elephant was quite a step up from immobilizing rhino, elephant were five to ten times larger (like moving up from driving a Toyota pickup truck to driving an 18 wheeler!), they were taller and could see considerably further than rhino and they were much smarter and calculating whereas by comparison a rhino was very limited in their physical capabilities and predictable. I had worked with large angus, shorthorn, Hereford and Charlaise bulls, Clydesdale horses, adult Asian elephants at the St. Louis Zoological Gardens and white and black rhino in South Africa so I was familiar with working with large animals and was not afraid. Now I had to learn to work with extremely aggressive animals that were 10 to 15 times larger so I was in a learning curve again. A miscalculation with an elephant meant certain death.

The actual process of tracking elephant was easier than tracking rhino; elephant were very noisy in their browsing and feeding – rhino were quiet and reclusive, elephant were very bold in coming to water holes during the daytime and were easier to see and tended to travel in large herds. You could escape a rhino charge by climbing up a tree or getting to the opposite side of a cactus thicket – there was no way to escape an elephant charge without having to take some drastic action – elephants can knock down or pull down trees!

We used one to three milligrams of Etorphine or M-99 (an opium derivative that was 25 times more potent than morphine) to immobilize adult elephant. Darts that were four to six inches long were filled with distilled water to act as a dispersant and the Etorphine added last. The needles attached to the darts were reinforced, barbed and had the diameter of a # 2 drafting pencil and about four inches long to ensure that it wouldn't brake or bounce off when it struck the elephant and to ensure complete delivery of the drug through the one inch thick skin.

After the 8,000 to 15,000 pound elephant was immobilized they were cold branded with branding irons super cooled in liquid nitrogen or dry ice to kill the pigment cells in their skin. After about two months the "brand" appeared as new non-pigmented cells that replaced the old cells. Heavy color-coded plastic sleeves were sewn snuggly around their tails and marine epoxy paint was used to paint numbers on the elephant's ears, shoulders and hips to monitor the elephant's movements until the "brand" developed. After the branding was done, measurements obtained, ticks collected and blood samples taken, an antidote (Nalorphine) was given to the elephant intravenously to counteract the effects of the immobilizing drug. The large garden hose sized ear veins that were used by the elephant to cool themselves were easily accessible to administer the drug. We would trot off down wind and squat in the shade of an acacia tree 25 - 50 yards away and wait to make sure the elephant got up.

Typically the elephant would start to increase their respiratory rate to normal within ten seconds and get up within one minute of being given the antidote. The elephant would take a minute or two to steady themselves, get their bearings, locate their herd and then take off on the run into the wind.

A standard form was given to each visitor in the park with a list of the symbols and numbers we had emblazoned on the elephant and we asked them to note any they observed, the elephant's location, if they were alone or with a herd, time of day of the sighting, etc. The visitors turned in the forms as they left the park for review and interpretation – we had a system.

The game rangers and scouts at the Wankie Reserve had never seen an elephant immobilized and I had to train them and inform them of what to expect while I was learning how to track and safely get within range of lone elephant and selected elephants in the middle of a herd.

The very first elephant to be immobilized was very, very exciting. A ranger, two game scouts and myself were tracking a lone adult bull to do a test run without the complications of a large herd to be concerned with. We wanted to confirm the potency of our supply of Etorphine and establish effective dosages and recovery times.

We were walking quietly into the wind following the steaming piles of manure on a narrow path through a forest observing broken and chewed, crushed and barkless twigs and browsing signs left by the 15,000-pound bull, when he suddenly and without warning stepped out onto the path and faced us from about 20 yards ahead. We froze in mid-step, the bull raised his trunk to sniff the air and "see" who we were; he rumbled a warning; we stayed frozen; he put his head down, curled his trunk under his chin, gave a blood curdling scream and charged!

The ranger and the two game scouts threw down their rifles and ran in the opposite direction; armed only with my modified 20 gauge shotgun tranquilizer gun and one loaded dart I stood my ground; the bull stopped at the ten yard mark gave a vigorous shake of his head flapping his ears throwing off dust and sand in the typical elephant challenge. He glared at me, screamed and came at me again – I raised the gun and fired the dart at the base of his trunk right between his eyes.

The dart struck and held; the bull looking dumbfounded at the insult inflicted upon him, a lot like a deer in the headlights, stopped suddenly only five yards away in a cloud of dust, leaves and twigs that rained down on me. He looked cross-eyed and examined the dart gently with the tip of his trunk while I loaded a second dart into the gun; he rumbled again, backed up, turned and ran off the path upwind crashing and plowing through the underbrush – he was now easier to track.

The ranger and game scouts trotted up to me laughing and shaking their heads, as they had never seen such a remarkable thing in their lives. They apologized for leaving me behind and declared that it wouldn't happen again because they now had faith in my skills and the power of the immobilizing drugs.

We found the bull several miles away obviously only partially tranquilized and in an odd position. He was standing, but not in a natural posture, he sagged backwards to an almost sitting position; because of the off balanced position and his effort to stay standing was a strain on his shoulders, he was quivering like a bowl full of jelly. When we approached him from behind he could only very, very slowly turn in our direction.

Attempts to pull the bull down by his tail were fruitless and rather than wasting another dart I gave him an additional 1 mg dose of Etorphine in his rump with a hand syringe; he collapsed on his side in five minutes and we went to work.

We immobilized almost fifty elephants over a three-month period and we learned many things including elephants in a herd were actually easier and safer to catch than lone individuals as they would rather stay with the herd rather than chase us. We became adept at the branding process and how to get the dry ice or liquid nitrogen from the nearest railhead or ranger station. We became very skilled and very confident in our ability to immobilize elephant and do our jobs.

On one occasion a less than typical reaction occurred after administrating the antidote to our elephant. The modest-sized female failed to get up even after 30 minutes following the administration of the antidote. Her respiration was good but she just made no attempt to get up.

I left my game scout behind with a shotgun and I ran back to the elephant to check her out. I found that I had left her large three-foot square ear that was used to give the antidote, flipped forward over her eye; normally the ear would be laid back in its normal position and her eye left uncovered.

Without much thought I flipped her ear back to the normal position and her eye immediately focused on me like the iris of a camera's zoom lens. I started running backwards as fast as I could as she lurched to her feet. This was a fully awake and a very angry female elephant. She curled her trunk under her chin, trumpeted the high-pitched warning given by elephants when danger is eminent and charged right at me.

She was gaining on me and I thought I was flying. With only steps to go before she caught up with me the game scout fired his shotgun. My shirt shredded and flew off and I felt like I was shot in the back with rock salt. In actuality the scout had shot the elephant in the front left foot with number 6 birdshot. The elephant stopped, looked at her foot, inspected it with her trunk, turned and ran off.

The scout had run towards me when he saw my predicament and was so close to me when he fired that the blast from the shotgun had ripped off my shirt and peppered me with sand and gunpowder.

After two years of rugged bush living in the Republic of South Africa and Southern Rhodesia (today called Zimbabwe) and first hand observations of the life, health, disease and death of hundreds of species of African wildlife large and small, I received a telegram from Marlin Perkins, of the Mutual of Omaha's Wild Kingdom fame, inviting me back to America.

Marlin wanted me to become a post-doctoral fellow at

Washington University as a wildlife pathologist. Because I believed that I was living the idyllic life, I wrote Marlin a polite "no thank you" note and set it on the mantel for mailing – a month later I realized that I hadn't sent the note. After much wrestling with the idea I relented and headed back to the U.S. – after all I was on a hunt for truth, and I already knew the EPIPHANY was universal in Africa!

It was time to take the hunt for truth back to the laboratory. It was time to take the hunt for truth back to America. It was time to take the truth found in the hunt to the people of America so it could be put to practical use. The EPIPHANY was the truth!

Marlin Perkins along with Dr. Barry Commoner, a botanist from Washington University in St. Louis, had gotten a $7.5 million dollar grant from the NIH to study pollution, disease and the world's ecology in animals, people and plants jointly with the Shaw's Botanical Gardens, Barnes Hospital and the Department of Biology of Washington University.

The 60's industrial mercury disaster in Mina Mata Bay in Japan that caused catastrophic birth defects in over 700 children set off scientific and political alarms all over the world. Science and governments were blind-sided and caught totally off guard. World paranoia over the pollution problem contributed to the divisions between conservationists and industry and between the young and the "establishment."

The combined facilities of the St. Louis Zoological Gardens, Shaw's Botanical Gardens and Washington University's school of biology and Barnes Hospital formed a new department called The Center for the Biology of Natural Systems. In addition to my pathology and clinical responsibilities in the zoo, the center provided an opportunity for me to become a post doctoral fellow and continue with my comparative pathology graduate studies and training in many different scientific disciplines in order to quickly integrate accumulated data.

The idea of the center was to trade data from many already completed research projects and leap frog from the research of one specialty to another to save time. Why do the research again at great cost of time and money when it had already been done by another scientific specialty? The project was like putting together the pieces of a great jig-saw puzzle from pieces collected individually from all over the world.

A second purpose of the center was to train a small group of new scientists who could effectively read the language of dozens of different sciences and solve problems quickly. We were trained by top researchers and noted professors in each field of appropriate science. We were placed in a crisis mode and urged to move forward quickly with our investigations. There didn't appear to be a lot of time, our government needed answers now!

My job as a postdoctoral fellow, the wildlife veterinarian and pathologist on the project was to do autopsies of captive animals dying in zoos around the United States. I was directed to look for a species of animal that was highly susceptible to the presence of even minute levels of pollution so we could use that species as an early warning signal or a "canary in the mine" to warn us of some impending environmental doom.

My direct academic supervisor was Dr. Malcolm Peterson, the chief anatomical pathologist at Barnes Hospital, Washington University, School of Medicine in St. Louis. Although I was already an accomplished and published comparative pathologist and well schooled in human disease at that point it was good to have the mentoring of a top human pathologist to further develop my skills in human pathology.

Unlike laboratory animals, pet animals and domestic species, zoo animals were not uniformly fed scientifically designed rations or diets in the 60s. Each zookeeper or curator tinkered with individual animals diets. Some based the zoo animal's diets on their own dietary preferences, some were based on myth and movies (i.e.- monkeys eat only fruit, lions only eat red meat, etc.) and some based diets on what fit into the zoo's budgets. As a result, the autopsies of zoo animals in the 1960's and 1970's were a treasure trove of nutritional deficiency diseases of every kind imaginable in every captive species.

Complete autopsies including the anatomical descriptions, organ shapes and weights, gross pathology, histological pathology, biochemistry, toxicology, microbiology, parasitology, a photographic museum and clinical histories were accumulated. After 12 years of performing autopsies on over 17,500 animals of more than 454 species of animals and more than 3,000 humans it became clear that pollution in the United States was not as insidious and widespread as originally feared. Pollution was on rare occasion a serious or catastrophic problem in local areas where mining, industry and agriculture failed to follow established rules and safeguards and contaminated the atmosphere, farmland and water sources.

The most profound finding in all of the more than 20,000 autopsies in both man and beast was that every animal and every human being that died of natural causes died of a nutritional deficiency disease! The findings just jumped out of the records – we weren't looking for nutritional deficiency diseases but there they were! The EPIPHANY again!

Diseases that were thought to be genetic or autoimmune in animals and humans were simple nutritional deficiency diseases. I now had hard evidence to answer the questions of a teenager – why did we give vitamins and minerals to animals and not ourselves. The EPIPHANY was now supported by hard data accumulated from hundreds of species of animals.

I cooperated with Ralston Purina animal feed division and Hills Packing Company, Science Diet Division to test and create many pellet and canned rations for various species of zoo animals. Species that had never lived to maturity in zoos began to live to old age; animals that never reproduced in zoos became fertile and began to breed and produce young; degenerative diseases (heart disease, goiter, arthritis, fibromyalgia, lupus, osteoporosis, Paget's disease, kidney stones, liver cirrhosis, aneurysms, diabetes) that were common in caged zoo animals and humans disappeared in zoo animals following proper supplementation of essential nutrients!

I wrote over 70 peer review and refereed articles for publication in veterinary and medical journals, contributed more than 15 chapters in eight multi-author text books on the subject and wrote a 1,000 page tome on comparative medicine and pathology which was published by the W.B. Saunders Company (the main publisher of medical texts) that is still found in medical school and veterinary school libraries today.

With the urging of Perkins, I developed a frozen and preserved tissue and organ bank at the St. Louis Zoo from material collected from the autopsies so that scientists from all over the world could have access to the tissue material collected from exotic species without having to kill additional individual animals.

I lectured to professional groups of clinical doctors, scientists and academics all over the world but found only too few who would embrace the EPIPHANY. They still believed that humans could get everything they needed from the basic four food groups and "the dangers of toxicity and overdose from nutritional supplements were too dangerous."

After working in many zoos throughout the United States I found myself in the Yerkes Regional Primate Research Center in Atlanta, Georgia doing service pathology for a wide variety of investigators. Some studied drug effects in primates, some studied nutrition, some studied behavior, some studied reproduction; some projects were simply designed to raise normal babies for other projects including NASA. A real plus was that the Center for Disease Control offices and laboratories were right across the street from Yerkes and I was able to participate in the weekly pathology conferences and continue to review and scrutinize human autopsies.

I did the pathology work on a variety of primates (i.e.- squirrel monkey, wooly monkey, rhesus monkey, baboon, chimpanzee, orangutang, etc.) that died of natural causes and on animals that were killed at the end of the study to determine if the study drugs or nutritional diseases had caused any tissue, organ or biochemical changes.

The most amazing finding occurred in November 1977 when I autopsied a six month old infant rhesus monkey that I diagnosed as having cystic fibrosis. Cystic fibrosis was supposed to be a genetic disease that occurred only in white people predominantly from middle and Eastern Europe. There had never been any cases of cystic fibrosis diagnosed in any animal nor had there ever been any laboratory animal model created for the study of cystic fibrosis (the reasons given for the failure to find the cure for cystic fibrosis).

After reviewing the medical reports on CF in humans I found that it had been diagnosed in Chinese, Africans, Eskimos, American Indians and that out of all the infants born to thousands of CF couples only one child had been diagnosed with CF. It was obvious from even a cursory review of existing cases that CF was not a genetic disease but rather a congenital defect caused by a maternal selenium deficiency. CF researchers were trying to put a square peg in a round hole!

On closer scrutiny it was obvious that the cystic fibrosis I had diagnosed in the rhesus monkey was created by a congenital nutritional deficiency of the trace mineral selenium and was re-creatable at will. We now had an animal model that could be used to study cystic fibrosis in humans.

My observations and diagnosis of CF in the monkey were quickly confirmed by the most respected of CF experts from the Johns Hopkins School of Medicine and the Chicago Lying In Hospital. I was commended in writing and given a raise in pay plus a letter of commendation for the discovery. To make a discovery that could help so many children and prevent such a terrible disease was a scientists dream. It was an exciting time.

In May of 1978, ten days after my wife, Josephine, was killed by an over aggressive chemotherapy program to treat Hodgkin's disease at the Grady Memorial Hospital in Atlanta, Georgia, I was terminated from my pathology post with only 24 hours notice because the proponents of the genetic theory of CF prevailed on Dr. Geoffrey Bourne, the director of Yerkes, to terminate me. I had unknowingly "kicked a hornet's nest" and had unwittingly become a potential financial competitor to a powerful genetic empire at the national level - I was only interested in the truth.

This negative knee jerk survival at all cost, sacrifice Wallach for the greater good of the genetic project reaction from the scientific community was another example of why there is so little progress being made for the elimination of certain diseases – egos and protection of research empires appear to be more important than truth.

I was now a widower with "four hungry children and a crop in the field." The children ranged in age from one year to 12 years. I had to care for them, find an income and try to keep the nutritional cause of CF research alive. I applied for jobs in my field, but I was "too hot to hire," the word had been put out by Dr. Bourne and official Yerkes mail, no one would risk losing funding to hire me. My productive 14-year comparative pathology career had ended suddenly with the added weight of the loss of my wife and the lone responsibility for the welfare of four kids.

In August of 1978 I began to lecture to the general public on the concepts of the EPIPHANY. Cystic Fibrosis family support groups were extremely interested in my research but powerless to get me back into the field of cystic fibrosis research.

After a series of adventures I found myself in Portland, Oregon teaching basic and clinical nutrition at the National College of Naturopathic Medicine in January 1979. A naturopathic physician or ND is trained and licensed as a primary care physician – including a full four – year basic science and four year medical curriculum and residency that allows the ND a scope of practice to do everything that an MD general practitioner can plus an ND is highly trained in clinical nutrition, Chinese medicine, herbal medicine and physical medicine. Although an ND can do surgery and write prescriptions they prefer to use conservative methods first – "first do no harm" is their motto!

I had come to a juncture – do I go to orthodox medical school and become an MD and fight (for perhaps the rest of my life) for the concept of preventing and curing disease with nutritional formulas or do I go a different direction and become an ND.

A long time friend and fellow Missouri veterinarian, Dr. John Troxel, convinced me that the orthodox research establishment would fight me forever – truth, he said was not the issue, it was the preservation of a multibillion dollar research empire that was at issue.

Medical doctors believed or at least preached that you could get all the vitamins, minerals and trace minerals that you needed from you basic four food groups. I had already tried to educate medical doctors for twenty years with no success. Naturopathic physicians already believed in the healing power of nutrition! Nutrition was a major approach that they used to heal their patients. I wouldn't have to convince them – they were already convinced. My dad always said, "The definition of insanity is that you keep doing the same thing over and over and expect a different outcome."

There was no longer a question of what to do – the choice became very clear. In fact there was no choice – I had to become a naturopathic physician so that I could legally treat humans! I had to grit my teeth, cut myself off from my long time associates and leave behind 20 years of orthodox biomedical and comparative medicine and pathology research, writing and teaching.
Robert Frost would describe my choice this way:

The Road Not Taken

Two roads diverged in a yellow wood,
And sorry I could not travel both
And be one traveler, long I stood
And looked down one as far as I could
To where it bent in the undergrowth;

Then took the other, as just as fair,
And having perhaps the better claim,
Because it was grassy and wanted wear
Though as for that the passing there
Had worn them really about the same,

And both that morning equally lay
In leaves no step had trodden black.
Oh, I kept the first for another day!
Yet knowing how way leads onto way,
I doubted if I should ever come back.

I shall be telling this with a sigh
Somewhere ages and ages hence;
Two roads diverged in a wood, and I –
I took the one less traveled by,
And that has made all the difference.

In 1979 I became a student again; as a result of my veterinary
training and graduate courses in comparative anatomy, medicine
and pathology I was able to start my residency as an advanced status student even as a freshman medical student. Under the supervision of licensed physicians I began to use basic veterinary nutritional formulas on human patients as a freshman. It was no real
surprise to me that the formulas designed to prevent, reverse and
cure diseases in animals worked just like a charm in humans! As
a junior medical student I purchased a small practice in Cannon
Beach, Oregon and hired two physicians to operate and build the
practice even before I graduated. I wanted to hit the ground running the day I graduated.

The purpose of my becoming an ND instead of an MD was to
be able to deliver the concept and benefits of the EPIPHANY to
human patients without having to again go through the frustration
of trying to convince skeptical doctors to believe and take action.
It was now obvious that if it was to be it was up to me! It was

obvious that medical doctors as a group weren't interested in preventing and curing diseases with nutritional formulas but that the general public was!

I realized that there was no law that required medical doctors to cure diseases in humans and end their suffering even when cures were available. There were no laws that required medical doctors to prevent diseases in humans even when there were preventions available.

The news of my patient successes in improving or reversing disease (i.e.- high blood pressure, type II diabetes, arthritis, osteoporosis, lupus, fibromyalgia, etc.) using the veterinary nutritional formulas (Dr. Wallach's Pig Arthritis Formula, etc.) spread quickly and people from over the world came to my little practice in Oregon. My patients told their friends and relatives, "If you're not happy with what your doctor's doing for you, go see Wallach, he'll treat you like a dog, but you'll get better!"

Chapter 12

Predators and Terrorists

"The only thing we have to fear is fear itself."

—Franklin D. Roosevelt

The strength of a nation is a reflection of the will of its people – the will to be self sufficient, the will to be free, the will to survive financially, the will to be healthy and the will to live healthfully long past 120!

To accomplish these goals of survival, long life and to flourish requires individual proactive output of effort and expenditure of time and resources for personal, family and the common good. Neither the government (city, county, state, federal) nor the American medical system has the interest, incentives or will because governments and the medical systems are made up of people with self-interest as their primary goal!

It is easy for a hungry, focused, dedicated vicious predator (lion, mugger or terrorist) to identify, isolate, terrorize and attack a naive, weak and unprepared individual victim. It is the mugger, terrorist or an armies dream to defeat a victim without having to fight and expose oneself to potential harm. Sun Tzu's *The Art of War* summarizes it best, "To subdue the enemy without fighting is the supreme excellence."

However, fear and terrorism by their very nature have not been successful as long-term weapons of occupation, they are the quick brush-block used by individuals to attack or mug individuals or armies to make war on the unprepared (WTC 9/11/01).

Fear and terror soon wear off - grazing animals, pigeons and people quickly go back to the business of daily life following an attack. If the perpetrators repeatedly follow up their initial terrorist attacks again and again, the survivors either flee or begin plotting a defense or better yet a counter attack (America's war on terrorism following the WTC attack on September 11, 2001; the Israeli defensive counter attack on Yasser Arafat's PLO compound following the constant suicide bombings and murder of Israelis by Al Aqsa in March 2002).

The American government, embattled with the Great Depression under President Hoover blocked oil sales to Japan as a non-military deterrent to Japanese expansion in the Pacific - the Japanese responded with the December 7, 1941 Pearl Harbor "sneak attack." The quick-footed Japanese already on a territory grabbing war footing quickly followed up their Pearl Harbor success with an invasion of the then American territory of Alaska.

The naive and initially unprepared Americans responded to the fear created by the Japanese invasion of Alaska (not the Pearl Harbor attack) by interning Japanese Americans on the west coast. Americans on the west coast reacted in a "do something" preemptory move to keep imagined Japanese sympathizers out of the predicted battle of the American west coast.

Large amounts of American energy, men and resources were diverted from the war in the Pacific to the home front to fight the Japanese in Alaska giving the Japanese time to expand unchecked in the Pacific and to invade the Philippine Islands.

The September 11, 2001 World Trade Center attack was not designed to be a pre-invasion blow for Al Qaeda, but rather the airplanes filled with thousands of gallons of high octane jet fuel were a poor mans atomic bomb, a bold terrorist act to destabilize the American domestic economy, create fear and hopefully cause the American people to demand a pull out of their protective positions in Saudi Arabia, Iraq and Israel – illustrated in Tom Clancy's *The Sum of all Fears* "kill one, frighten 10,000."

After all, the truck bomb killing of 230 marines in Lebanon and the killing of 18 special forces rangers in Somalia resulted in an almost immediate American withdrawal from these foreign wars each time – the lesson was "kill American soldiers and the Americans will run home."

The WTC attack was a predictable chess move – kill Americans in large numbers and they will fold and withdraw was the repeated lesson of previous attacks.

The firing of Tomahawk cruise missiles by then U.S. President Clinton into Afghanistan following the 1998 terrorists bombing attacks on American embassies in Africa was considered by the terrorist a generic, weak and impotent response - designed only to impress Americans at home.

The simultaneous hijacking of four commercial airliners on September 11, 2001 to use as guided missiles against the World Trade Center twin towers, the Pentagon and a fourth American icon (presumably the White House) was extremely creative and in their minds a logical next move by the Muslim fundamentalist terrorist – after all, what would the Americans do, launch a Tomahawk cruise missile into the Afghanistan desert again?

There was a longtime effort in planning and a successful worldwide conspiracy by multiple terrorist "cells" that resulted in significant American civilian casualties (3,000 killed and 2,400 injured in the WTC attacks), injured the American economy, destroyed physical assets of American business (World Trade Center) and the American military (the Pentagon), destroyed American confidence and yet our government's high priced intelligence system was absolutely blind sided.

Pentagon personnel watched the WTC attacks on TV for almost an hour without sending up an umbrella of military protection for itself or other government assets.

Therefore it is evident that we cannot expect or depend on our government or medical systems to protect each individual against street muggers or terrorist attacks of any kind. It is then absolutely essential that each individual understand and know how to protect themselves and their loved ones from disease and various levels and types of attacks– to do this we must learn to be observant, educate and arm ourselves with basic health, nutrition, self treatment and survival knowledge.

Self and Home Defense:

Martial arts are great for the novice and the black belt level expert defending themselves and loved ones against unarmed muggers and thieves, however, intense training, motivation, surprise and a "take action" attitude can overcome overwhelming odds.

Only two weeks after arriving in the U.S. as an exchange scholar microsurgeon with Harvard Medical School, Ma Lan (an expert in oriental martial arts) was mugged. Two teenagers, armed with "Saturday night specials" surrounded and accosted her loudly demanding that she give them her purse. She was startled, but didn't understand their demands for her purse on that cold winter night in Boston. They moved into range as one of the muggers grabbed her purse and the other grabbed her long black hair and laughed – big mistake.

Ma Lan grabbed the gun and the wrist of the first would-be mugger bending it backward to produce extreme pain (he dropped to his knees and dropped his gun), Ma Lan straight kicked the second mugger in the groin (he hesitated because the first mugger was now between him and Ma Lan), she quickly turned on the second hapless mugger with a straight arm punch to the jaw – it was over in seconds. Ma Lan was motivated and took action – she had survived the Cultural Revolution in China and was not about to be killed by teenagers with guns only two weeks after arriving in the U.S.

Invasion of one's home by an invading army or terrorist is highly unlikely in America; however, muggings on the street and home invasions by thieves, burglars and kidnappers are common. Dead bolts, alarms, panic buttons, multiple phones, closed garages, dogs, pepper spray and baseball bats are all part of a basic home security system.

When an armed intruder gets into your home the average person will either have to run and evade the intruder or stand your ground and use deadly force in defense. Guns for home defense are an option that each person must weigh for themselves, as there are multiple safety responsibilities if you keep guns in the house:

- Handguns are the top choice for home security - they should be full size and designed with maximum knockdown capacity (i.e.- .22 magnum, .25 ACP caliber, .38 caliber, 9 mm, .45 caliber, .357 magnum). Handguns require lots of practice to assure accuracy and rapid proficiency in an emergency.
- Shotguns should have a short barrel, pump-loading action, with man killing 00 "buckshot" shells that contain nine .30 caliber pellets per shell.
- Rifles have the advantage of being light weight plus the availability of multiple preloaded magazines (i.e.-.22 caliber, .223 caliber, .30.06).

Truck and car bombs:

Truck and car bombs are considered by experts to be the first line of easily available terrorist weapons. The first known and recorded "truck bomb" was detonated by Israeli nationalist in Jerusalem on July 22, 1946. A truck loaded with high explosives and a delay fuse was driven into the courtyard of the King David Hotel and abandoned by the driver. The resulting 91 British deaths and massive hotel damage ushered in the words "truck bomb" into the English dictionary.

The truck and car bomb, vehicle delivered explosive and

incendiary, has been a basic tool of terrorists worldwide ever since the King David Hotel bombing. A truck bomb in Beirut, Lebanon driven by a Hezbollah suicide terrorist killed 241 U.S. marines while they slept in 1983.

The Murrah Federal Building in Oklahoma City was ripped in half in 1995, killing 168 people, by a simple fertilizer bomb in a rented truck. The first World Trade Center bombing in 1993 was a truck bomb as were the 1994 Khobar Towers bombing in Saudi Arabia that killed 19 U.S. servicemen and the U.S. embassy bombings in East Africa in 1998 that killed more than 200.

The FBI continues to investigate truck-driving schools, specifically reviewing 2.5 million licenses issued to carry hazardous material because of the risk of such drivers hauling materials that could be used as bombs. A group of 25 Arab men trained and licensed to drive big rigs had raised the red flag because the method that they used to obtain their training was almost identical to that used by the September 11, 2001 hijackers to get pilot training.

The 25 men attended a big rig driving school in Colorado, each paid cash and none of them looked for work after getting their certificate.

Dr. Stefan H. Leader, a security analyst says that a common terrorist tactic with truck and car bombs "is the use of two devices placed close to each other, with the second device set to go off a few minutes after the first." Dr. Leader says, " The first explosion is intended to attract security personnel to the scene; the second is intended to kill and injure them. This tactic has been used by Islamic terrorists in Israel and by the Provisional Irish Republican Army in Northern Ireland and the United Kingdom. It was used for the first time in the United States in January of 1997 at the Atlanta abortion clinic bombing."

The best defense against truck and car bombs is not mechanical barriers, but rather group awareness – each person is part of the defense system of our towns, state and country. You should contact security authorities if you observe:

- A truck or car parked in a restricted zone.
- An unusual truck or car parked in a loading zone.
- A stranger arguing with security employees.
- A person running from a parked or abandoned truck or car.

Vehicle security and safety tips include:

- Plan your trip in detail, have a mental picture of the route; don't stop to read maps.
- Park in area with security lights or inside of a garage.
- Weak hand grasps keys and flashlight allowing dominant hand to be free for defense.
- Use mouth to hold and aim small penlight leaving both hands free.
- Check the underside and motor compartment of your vehicle daily.
- Learn the basics of car and truck computers and electrical systems.
- Use an angled mirror on a pole to look at your vehicle's underside.
- Check under car's seat (especially driver's) before entering car.
- Call 911 if suspicious – do not deal with unusual problems by yourself.
- Use your vehicle as a weapon if you come under attack by muggers, carjackers or terrorists.
- When waiting in vehicles, park close to lights, walls, fences and buildings.
- Be rude when your life is at risk.
- Do not thumb a ride or pick up hitchhikers or "victims" who

can be "bait."

- Watch out for carjackers or terrorists dressed as police or security forces.

Suicide bombers:

Suicide bombers combine the terror effect of bombing unexpected targets (usually civilian) with a variety of means to deliver the bomb in person including buses, trucks, cars, airplanes, boats, motorcycles, packages, brief cases, cell phones, dogs, horses and their own bodies (coats, vests, belts, shoes, etc.).

Suicide bombers will look out of place like a "fish out of water," they will often times be nervous, sweating and agitated. Suicide bombers are almost always young men between the ages of 18 and 35 (young women are more and more being used as suicide bombers in the middle east) and are almost always Arabic, Asian or African Muslims. They will buy one-way tickets on public transportation with cash, and have little or no checked baggage.

A typical example of a would-be suicide bomber is Richard Reid (aka: Abdel Rahim), a small-time British thug who converted to Islam in prison and was lured into the Al Qaeda Muslim extremist group in 1995. With no apparent means of income or baggage, Reid traveled back and forth from Pakistan, Egypt, France, Israel, the Netherlands, and various countries in North Africa before his final travel leg from Paris to Miami.

Reid, 28 years old, looked unkempt, had no baggage, held a newly issued English passport and attempted to buy a one-way ticket from Paris to Miami with cash. On his first try he was retained and searched because of his suspicious profile; he missed his flight so American Airlines paid for his room and board and again despite objections of fellow passengers he successfully boarded the Paris to Miami flight 63 the next morning.

At the halfway point between Paris and Miami, Reid, still sitting in his assigned seat over the plane's starboard wing and fuel tank, struck a match in an attempt to light a fuse protruding from explosives in the heel of one of his sneakers.

An analysis of Reid's explosives showed them to be a mix of the volatile TATP (triacetone triperoxide) and the more stable and powerful PETN (pentaerythritol tetranitrate). It is believed that the TATP can easily be made from a recipe of common household chemicals and is used to set off the more stable PETN. The PETN is a commercial grade explosive considerably more powerful than TNT and is a component of Semtex, a Czech-made plastic explosive.

An alert stewardess, who smelled the sulfur fumes released by the match and heard the screams from Reid's fellow passengers tried to grab the match and shoe from Reid.

Reid, who is six foot four inches tall, vigorously resisted attempts to restrain him by the stewardess and fellow passengers, so they began throwing water on him and his matches. Reid was finally overwhelmed by a half dozen passengers and tied up and drugged for the remainder of the trip.

What if Reid would have gone into the toilet, disarmed the smoke alarm and then attempted to set off his bomb away from the prying eyes of his fellow passengers? Again, individual action by a flight attendant and willing passengers saved the day for American Airlines flight 63 from certain disaster from the would-be suicide bomber as there were no sky marshals aboard!

Nuclear, chemical and biological warfare:

In the case of nuclear, chemical and biological warfare simple information can be the difference between life and death for one-self, loved ones, neighbors and workmates. Knowledge is power – being prepared is power!

Learn basic survival skills. Learn how to use a compass; carry a cell phone; carry a whistle; learn methods of purifying water (10 drops of chlorine bleach per pint and leave the water set for 24 hours before using); learn how to track a human or animals; learn how to catch small game animals for food; learn first aid; learn how to prevent hypothermia and heat stroke; learn how to use landscaping plants as food; grow an indoor garden with tomatoes and other vegetables; learn how to identify and use herbs as plant medicines; learn how to produce energy from solar, wind and hydropower.

Water filters with carbon block elements can remove particulate matter, asbestos, atrazine, benzine, MTBE, lead and other chemicals but are not considered dependable for removing bacteria or viruses.

Learn simple self-defense. Learn how to use a pen, pencil, keys, screwdriver, hammer, book, thermos, hands, elbows and feet as weapons. Take martial arts courses. Learn how to handle, clean, repair and shoot firearms. Confidence and survival skills are power!

Terrorism, though ultimately unsuccessful long-term can have a short-term devastating effect on individual people. Some psychologists say that concerns about the emotional effects caused by bombing large municipalities encouraged the British government to give in to Adolph Hitler before World War II – one military general felt if London was bombed it would become a "Bedlam," the historical English mental hospital famous for being a large single cage full of mentally ill people with chaotic and bizarre behavior.

Despite losing 20,000 civilians killed to Nazi V1 and V2 rocket and bombing attacks during the 1940 – 41 "blitz" on London the British people did not succumb to mass panic or surrender because of the will and motivational skills of one man – Sir Winston Churchill. One person can make a difference. "Never! Never! Never surrender!"

Nuclear Devices:

Nuclear attacks on metro, military and historical sites are more likely today than during the Cold War as terrorist groups are men without a country and they have shown by their attack on the World Trade Center they have no morals or target limits.

Following the September 11, 2001 attack on the WTC the United Nations' International Atomic Energy Agency, an international watchdog agency warns that terrorist may steal radioactive medical or industrial waste materials to build "dirty bombs" that will be aimed at airports, subways, train stations, sporting events and other public places.

There are growing concerns over the safety of nuclear power plants, fueled by the reports of Pakistan detaining two prominent nuclear scientists linked to the Al Qaeda network. The federal Nuclear Regulatory Commission (NRC) continues to ask the 103 nuclear plants nationwide to keep security at its highest level.

"Everyone concurs now that terrorists have no qualms about what targets they go after," says NRC spokesperson Melisa Fleming. In addition to the theft of radioactive medical and industrial material, the agency's concerns center on:

- Nuclear plants. Sabotage of a reactor could lead to a Chernobyl-sized disaster.
- Nuclear fuel. Theft or diversion of plutonium or uranium could be a technique used by terrorist to create a nuclear bomb. Approximately 18 pounds of plutonium would be needed to construct a nuclear bomb.
- Suitcase bombs. There is continued concern over the sale or theft of suitcase-size nuclear devices designed by the Soviet Union.
- Traditional nuclear weapons. Collapse of a nuclear power (i.e.-Pakistan) could put existing weapons in the hands of terrorists.

Since 1993, the NRC has confirmed 376 cases of illegal sales or stolen radioactive materials. In 1987, Cesium-137 stolen from a medical clinic in Brazil killed four people.

Plutonium is ounce for ounce the most toxic substance on earth. Rather than build a conventional nuclear device that may be hard to transport and deliver, terrorists can choose to build a casing of plutonium around a truck bomb and unlike chemical agents plutonium contamination remains radioactive for more than 20 years.

A Newsweek magazine interview with CIA sources revealed that, "Al Qaeda had already obtained black-market cesium-137 and cobalt-60, and might have already experimented with "dirty bomb" dispersing devices prior to the September 11, 2001 World Trade Center attack."

Exploded with dynamite or other easily gotten explosives, a radioactive "dirty bomb" could kill thousands and injure tens of thousands through radiation poisoning – the terror factor alone would be enormous. "A terrorist with a little technical know-how and 20 pounds of smuggled plutonium could make a bomb powerful enough to completely destroy a major city. That's what we should be worried about," said a Pentagon spokesman in a New York Times interview May 13, 1996.

Like all risks, if you know what they are and how to deal with them their danger diminishes. There are people who live near nuclear power plants and don't realize that it is there. Get state, regional and national maps and clearly mark the locations of power plants, decommissioned nuclear plants (i.e.- Rocky Flats, Denver, CO) and nuclear wastes dumps (Nevada). Keep a 72-hour water and food reserve, portable radio, batteries, and a complete first aid kit; keep a "bail out" kit on hand to quickly throw in your car and go!

Have various escape routes mapped out in advance taking into account wind patterns. Get a radiation-monitoring device (remember the water salesman in Mel Gibson's Road Warrior movie Thunder Dome – Gibson tested the water and found it to be radioactive and didn't buy) – a CDV-715 radiation meter can be purchased from a surplus store for $250 dollars. If you live near nuclear sources of any type keep a store of potassium iodide on-hand, which can lower the risk of thyroid cancer following radiation exposure.

Chemical Agents:

Chemical and biological agents can be delivered in smoke (burning boats, cars, houses, grass fires, forest fires, wood piles, etc.), mists, aerosols, spray, dusts and explosions. Mere contact of drops of jelly, dust or smoke on exposed skin can cause symptoms of general paralysis, respiratory paralysis, choking, lung hemorrhaging, anemia and death.

Chemical warfare can be divided into several categories. Chemical agents can be dispersed as true gasses or solids and liquids dispersed as aerosols:

Pepper spray - is used by police or individual citizens (key chain dispensers) for close-up self-defense and to incapacitate an attacker. Causes severe burning sensation, irritation and production of mucus and tears in eyes, nose and throat – on rare occasions overdoses can be fatal when irritated throat membranes swell and cause death by respiratory obstruction and choking.

Tear gas is commonly used to temporarily incapacitate individuals or disperse large crowds. CS is the most commonly used tear gas for riot control around the world. CS causes severe irritation of eyes, nose and throat resulting in tearing, coughing and choking – large inhaled doses can cause death and delivery canisters can cause fires.

Fatal aerosols, gases and jellies:

Nerve agent: Nerve agents are clear colorless liquids. As a rule of thumb G agents are highly volatile and will degrade and become harmless within a few days. By contrast V agents are dangerous for weeks. Common characteristics of nerve agents are that they are extremely toxic and produce rapid incapacitation and death. The nerve agent is used as a liquid, aerosol or gas and is highly effective in causing death following skin contact or inhalation

Low doses of nerve agent produce salivation, nasal mucus discharge, angina, constricted pupils, fatigue, headache, nausea, hallucinations and slurred speech. High doses of nerve agent produce convulsions, coma, muscular paralysis, respiratory failure and death.

Protection and treatment for contact with nerve agents include physical protection (protective suits, masks, shelters, evacuate); medical protection (pre-exposure treatment drugs and herbs); detection (alarm, monitoring, identification, all-clear); and surface decontamination (personal and equipment) with lots of soapy water.

Mustard gas was first used as a weapon of mass destruction in WW I, it produces blisters at point of contact and can result in fatalities if inhaled.

In the 1930s organophosphates known as **G agents** were initially formulated by the German pharmaceutical giant IG Farben as a pesticide and were immediately recognized and researched for their military value.

Tabun (O-ethyl dimethylamidophosphorylcyanide or GA) was the first of the organophosphates; 12,000 tons were produced by Germany for use during WW II.

Sarin (isopropyl methylphosphonofluoridate or GB), the second organophosphate gas was developed in 1938 just prior to the U.S. entering WW II; it was designed to cause respiratory failure. In 1995 a Japanese cult injured thousands and killed 12 people in a Tokyo subway with Sarin gas: The gas was brought into the subway in inflated bags and balloons that were punctured with umbrella points to release the gas.

Soman (pinacolyl methylphosphonofluoridate or GD) was the third organophosphate chemical agent developed in 1944 as a nerve agent. The Soviet Union began serious production and stockpiling of Soman in 1997 and is thought to be in the hands of Iraq.

GF (Cyclohexyl methylphosphonofluoridate) is used as a gas or aerosol.

VX (O-ethyl S-diisopropylaminomethyl methylphosphonothiolate) is used as a gas or aerosol.

Choking agent:

Phosgene is considered the most dangerous of the choking agents - it produced 80% of all chemical warfare deaths in WW I.

Blood agent:

Hydrogen cyanide is used worldwide in the industrial production of acrylic polymers and therefore easy to obtain – it was used extensively by Iraq during the Iraq-Iran war.

Biological Agents:

Biological agents include viruses and bacteria and the toxins they produce, they are simple to produce and spread via aerosol, sprays, smoke, water, food and unlike chemical warfare they can be transmitted from one individual to another in varying degrees and therefore can terrorize and infect large populations far away from the site of initial release – "I will show you fear in a handful of dust" in *The Waste Land* by T.S. Eliot.

Scientists currently estimate that 1,500 "germ banks" – from Bangkok to Buenos Aires, Paris to Perth – keep dozens of strains of *Bacillus anthracis* and millions of other potentially dangerous bacteria on hand for "research purposes." Prices of biological agents vary from country to country.

> **Ricin** is a highly toxic phytochemical extracted from castor bean (*Ricinus communis*) oil. The castor bean has been used for medicinal purposes for over 4,000 years, yet two beans are enough to kill an adult. Ricin, a highly toxic protein found in the castor bean is used as a water or food borne poison. Ricin poisoning causes gastritis, nausea, vomiting, abdominal cramps, purging, hemorrhagic diarrhea, kidney failure, uremia, liver disease and death.

Bacterial toxins:

> **Botulinum** toxin produced by *Clostridium botulinum*, which causes paralysis and death, symptoms appear in 24 to 36 hours after exposure; initial symptoms are similar to those of food poisoning and can include blurred vision, difficulty in swallowing and speaking – it is odorless and tasteless and can be delivered in food or water supplies. On a gram for gram comparison, botulinum toxin is the most potent poison on earth – one pound of concentrated botulinum toxin properly dispersed could kill one billion people. The largest natural outbreak of botulism in the United States occurred in 1977 when 59 people fell ill after eating a contaminated batch of jalapeno peppers.

Infectious agents:

> **Smallpox virus** or *Variola major* killed more than 500 mil-

lion people during the 20th century alone. The smallpox virus has devastating potential because the disease has been eliminated from the world as a natural infection in 1977, there are no known treatments or cures and vaccinations were stopped worldwide in 1980 – previously vaccinated individuals have all but lost their original acquired immunity for lack of booster shots, and are dying from old age.

In 1980 all countries were then required to turn in their small-pox virus reserves and experimental stores of virus to the World Health Organization for official cataloging and destruction. The only remaining reserves were to be held and closely guarded by the CDC in Atlanta, Georgia and the Vector Biological Warfare Laboratories in Russia as a hedge against some future outbreak of smallpox. It is currently believed, however, that several maverick groups have access to smallpox virus and have the will to use it as a bio-weapon.

Several nations continue to endanger the world by biological and chemical weapons research including:

1) **Iraq** – When UN inspectors arrived in Iraq after the end of the 1991 Persian Gulf War Baghdad denied it possessed a biological warfare program. In July of 1995, the head of Iraq's weapons development programs, Hussein Kamal, a son-in-law of President Saddam Hussein defected.

This forced Iraq to admit it kept a cache of 8,500 liters of anthrax spores and 12,000 liters of botulism toxin. The UN inspectors uncovered and destroyed hardware used for large-scale anthrax processing at al-Hakam outside of Baghdad. "The precise status of Iraq's chemical and biolog-ical weapons programs is unknown because of that coun-try's efforts since 1991 to conceal the full extent of its pro-hibited activities," Johnathan Tucker of the Monterey Institute of International Studies told a U.S. Senate hearing in November of 2001. "It appears likely, however, that Iraq has rebuilt key elements of its chemical and pharmaceutical production infrastructure that were destroyed during the Gulf War and by [UN inspectors]," he added.

2) **North Korea** – A 1993 Russian intelligence report claims that North Korea is performing military research on pathogens such as anthrax, cholera, bubonic plague and smallpox and that weapons are being tested on island facilities. "North Korea probably has the ability to produce limited quantities of traditional infectious biological – weapon agents and toxins," a 1996 U.S. Department of Defense report claims.

3) **Iran** – In 1988, Iran's parliamentary speaker, Hashemi Rafsanjani, said, "chemical and biological weapons are a poor man's atomic bombs and can be easily produced. We should at least consider them for our defense." Citing intelligence officials, the Times of London has reported that Iran has conducted extensive research on agents such as anthrax, plague, foot-and-mouth disease and biotoxins.

4) **Libya** – Libya has been accused of developing chemical weapons in Tarhunah, a facility dug into hundreds of yards of mountain rock. "Libya has a biological-weapons program, but the country lacks the scientific and technical base to produce agents on a large scale, limiting its program to the research and development stage," General Wesley Clark, then commander in chief of the U.S. European Command, said in 2000.

5) **Sudan** – in 1998, the U.S. fired cruise missiles at a Khartoum pharmaceutical plant, saying that it manufactured a nerve-gas ingredient. There have been no public reports until November of 2001 that Sudan has developed a biological weapon.

The real danger is not that maverick nations will launch a biological attack directly against the United States or other western nations but rather that militant factions within them might purchase or hijack the technology.

Most baby boomers, their children and grandchildren have not been vaccinated against smallpox and they represent highly susceptible populations. One case of smallpox in the world today would create a global emergency.

Smallpox virus has an incubation period of seven to 14 days and is highly infectious and transmissible killing 30% of those infected and incapacitating the balance – infected populations would begin to show symptoms (fever, headache, nausea, etc), debilitation and death without knowing that they had been attacked two weeks earlier!

The Chinese invented inoculation for smallpox by putting smallpox scabs in the noses of children. Black American slaves survived smallpox outbreaks at a higher rate than their white owners by inoculating themselves with pus from smallpox pustules of victims.

White colonial doctors refused to employ the concept of inoculation as a preventative for smallpox and condemned it as an unclean practice until 1776 when a small town English physician by the name of Edward Jenner used cow pox (*Variola minor*) as a vaccination to prevent and eliminate smallpox infections in his village.

People with blood groups B and O have a greater natural resistance to the smallpox virus than do people with blood type A. Pizzaro and 168 Spanish soldiers defeated a war-hardened army of 80,000 Aztecs and Incas in 1526 at the battle of Cajamarca. Because the Spanish were carriers of the smallpox virus – the nation of 8 million Aztecs and Incas were decimated by 95% prior to Pizzaro's arrival because they had no cultural experience with small pox.

The emperor Atahuallpa and his army had come to Cajamarca to finish the decisive battle in their civil war – this war left the

Incas divided and vulnerable. Pizzaro rapidly recognized the divisions and exploited them. The cause of the civil war was that an epidemic of smallpox, spreading ahead of the Spanish settlers in Panama and Columbia, had killed the Inca Emperor Huayna Capac and most of his court in 1526; and then smallpox killed his immediate heir, Ninan Cuyuchi.

Those deaths precipitated a palace revolution for the throne between Atahuallpa and his half brother Huascar. If it had not been for the smallpox epidemic Pizzaro would have faced a healthy and united Inca Empire with one million warriors and the course of history in South America may have been different.

The British successfully used smallpox as a weapon during the French and Indian wars by distributing virus infected blankets to the Indian allies of the French.

Because there is no cure for the disease, smallpox is the ultimate bio-weapon and bio-terrorism tool.

Q – fever is caused by *Coxiella burnettii*, a rickettsial organism that produces flu-like symptoms, high fever, chills, tremors, diarrhea, congestive heart failure, hallucinations, facial pain and throbbing headaches - one out of a hundred infected individuals will die. Rickettsiae are organisms that are highly infectious (one organism can produce a clinical infection) and they behave like viruses in that they use the host cell's replicating mechanisms yet are susceptible to tetracycline antibiotic treatment.

Controlled military field tests of Q – fever rickettsiae showed that the organisms could remain infective and travel as far as 50 miles downwind after dispersal as a liquid spray from an airplane.

Anthrax (*Bacillus anthracis*) is a life threatening bacterial infection that can be delivered by aerosol (dust, spray, smoke, etc.), mail, food or water. Early symptoms can occur within 3 to 10 days following exposure (delayed infection can occur months after exposure) and can include deep skin ulcers, pimples, skin rashes, flu-like symptoms, fever, shock, meningitis, respiratory failure and death to 80 - 100% of those infected via the pulmonary route if not quickly and properly treated – considerably less transmissible than smallpox virus, however, anthrax pulmonary infection can on rare occasion be transmissible via coughing and sneezing.

Patients infected with anthrax often times show an initial improvement (known as the anthrax honeymoon) as their immune system tries to defend the host, but death can follow soon after the dead bacteria's release of toxins.

The infectious spores can survive in the environment for more than 40 years. There are 1,200 known varieties and strains of anthrax bacteria that can be identified by DNA testing.

Anthrax occurs naturally as an endemic infection in American livestock. Vaccination of livestock for anthrax is common in certain areas of the U.S.

The first serious human anthrax outbreak in the United States was reported in the Arms Textile Mill in Manchester, New Hampshire in 1957 following the importation of spore-contaminated goatskins from Pakistan.

Six hundred of the employees of the Arms Textile Mill were vaccinated against anthrax in 1955 in a military experiment. In 1957 nine of the unvaccinated employees came down with "wool sorters disease" or the skin form of anthrax from a natural exposure. The building was closed, demolished, burned to the ground and the remaining bricks were ordered buried for 2,000 years.

Nine years later an employee from across the parking lot from the Arms Textile Mill came down with inhalation anthrax – stray anthrax spores had survived mans best efforts to disinfect the area.

The Soviet Union had an anthrax disaster in April of 1979 when an army anthrax production plant blew up creating a spore cloud that killed thousands of farm animals and people in a number of villages downwind of the plant. It was estimated that a trillion anthrax spores or a total weight of one gram was released into the environment. The initial anthrax cluster occurred in the village of Sverdlosk where hundreds fell ill and 66 died from pulmonary anthrax. Villages as far down wind as 30 miles from the production facility recorded anthrax deaths.

Between 1990 and 1993 the Aum Shinrikyo cult in Japan released anthrax spores into large crowds four times yet no one was diagnosed with clinical anthrax or died. Several maverick countries are studying and producing anthrax as biological weapons and they are thought to have large stockpiles including Iraq, Iran, North Korea, Sudan and Russia.

On Tuesday, September 18, 2001 a small release of anthrax spores was delivered by mail (post marked from Trenton, New Jersey) in West Palm Beach Florida, killing one mail room employee and exposing 770 employees of a publishing facility – the isolated anthrax known as the Ames strain was developed in Iowa during the 1950s for research and widely shared with investigators around the world.

Anthrax spore releases next occurred by mail on Tuesday October 9, 2001 (post marked Trenton, New Jersey) in New York at the ABC and NBC news offices exposing several people including a seven month old child of an ABC employee that visited one day at the end of September and became infected with the cutaneous form of anthrax.

A highly refined weaponized anthrax release occurred on Tuesday October 9, 2001 by mail to the offices of senate minority leader Tom Daschle, D-S.D. where more than 20 of his staffers were exposed when the delivery envelope was opened. The two grams of highly refined anthrax spores had the potential to kill two million Americans.

By the end of October 2001 four Americans had died of pulmonary anthrax, and a dozen more were exposed to anthrax; the cutaneous form of anthrax was diagnosed in dozens of Americans and more than 10,000 postal, FDA and news agency workers from New York, New Jersey, Maryland, Florida, Missouri, Indiana and Washington, DC were being treated with preemptory antibiotics following discovery of anthrax spores on computers and postage machines.

Two of the first four to die from pulmonary anthrax were postal workers from the Trenton, New Jersey post office. One of the men called 911 the night before he died and the 911-operater recorded his last words. He believed he was infected with anthrax and exhibited many of the symptoms of pulmonary anthrax, yet his doctor told him, "You probably have a case of the flu, take plenty of fluids and get in bed." He died the next morning from pulmonary anthrax. This terrible incident is another example of how depending on doctors can kill you – if this man had penicillin and treated himself he would have lived!

In an unrelated case 41-year-old Kathy Nguyen, a New York hospital worker died of pulmonary anthrax in November of 2001 with no obvious avenue of infection.

The last known fatal anthrax case following the Trenton, New Jersey attacks was a 94-year-old Oxford, Connecticut woman, Ottile Lundgren – the DNA strain of the anthrax bacteria that killed her November 21, 2001 was the same strain that caused the other fatal infections. Although test on the mail found in her home were negative, the most likely source of the anthrax spores that killed Ottilie Lundgren was a cross contaminated birthday card from her U.S. Senator sent from Washington D.C.

FBI investigators said they were tracking purchases of the milling equipment necessary to weaponize anthrax spores. They are also curious about whether the mailing of the spore carrying letters on Tuesdays - September 18th and October 9th could indicate something about the terrorists work schedule or a window of time access to a microbiology laboratory.

Authorities believe the attacker is a loner type disenchanted male much like the reclusive Unabomber. Ted Kaczynski – because he was careful enough to make his own bomb parts (he even tooled his own screws from wire) and ride 1,500 miles one way on a bus to mail bombs to his victims – it took 18 years and a brother turning him in to authorities to close the case.

It is estimated that 2,500 to 55,000 spores measuring one to five microns each are required to cause a pulmonary infection. Unknown to the CDC microbiologist and perhaps even the bio-terrorists themselves, anthrax spores can pass through the paper pores in a tape-sealed envelope. It is estimated that 200 pounds of crude anthrax bacteria or spores released upwind of Washington D.C. could kill 3 million people.

Plague (*Yersinia pestis*) is a life threatening bacterial infection that can be delivered by aerosol (dust, spray, smoke, etc.), food or water; however, it is typically spread by contaminated biting insects such as fleas and bedbugs and is highly contagious. In the 14th Century one third of the European population and 13 million Chinese died from the "Black Death." Between 1980 and 1994 18,739 naturally occurring cases of plague were diagnosed worldwide in a total of 20 countries. Endemic sylvatic plague causes a few reports of illness and death each year in those tourists visiting prairie dog villages in the southwestern states of the U.S.

Humans are open to exposure and infection by three different routes and types of plague: bubonic plague, typified by swollen lymph nodes known as "buboes" in the inguinal and axillary folds; septicemic plague known as a "blood poisoning"; and pneumonic plague causing pneumonia that can be transmitted by aerosols from blood, a sneeze, cough or tears.

Early symptoms occur in one to six days following exposure and include high fever, coughing, respiratory failure and death.

Without prompt antibiotic treatment, bubonic plague kills 50% of those infected; untreated septicemic and pneumonic plague would be 100% fatal.

During World War II the Japanese air dropped tons of fleas infected with *Yersinia pestis* on Chinese villages resulting in the deaths of tens of thousands of peasants from plague used as a biological weapon.

Salmonella, Shigella, Escherichia coli and **staphylococcus** are low grade debilitating (vomiting and diarrhea) but potentially life threatening (dehydration and bacterial toxins) bacterial infections recognized by the general public as "food poisoning."

In 1984 zealous devotees of the Bhagwan Shree Rajneesh in Antelope, Oregon contaminated the towns water supply, drinking water glasses of county officials and the salad bars of ten restaurants including Shakey's Pizza in The Delles, Oregon with a *Salmonella typhimurium* bacterial slurry; they put it in blue-cheese dressing, coffee creamers and potato salad for the purpose of seizing control of the county government by incapacitating officials and opposition voters. No one died in the bio-terror attack but 751 people were struck with nausea, severe diarrhea, chills, fever, and dizziness.

A complete criminal investigation showed that the Bhagwan's followers had concocted complex plots to kill or infect 11 people on an "enemies" hit list including the U.S. attorney, several county officials, a follower who had sued the cult and a reporter from the Oregonian newspaper.

The scary part of the investigation was that the cult's staff successfully ordered several species of disease and death causing bacteria (i.e.- *Salmonella typhimurium* 14028, S. *paratyphi*, *Franscella tularensis*, *Enterobacter cloacae*, *Neisseria gonorrhoeae* and *Shigella dysenteriae*) from the American Type Culture Collection in 1984 and 1985.

In 1986 a natural outbreak of salmonellosis in a Chicago

milk processing plant caused 17,000 confirmed clinical cases.

In 1987 a CDC confirmed outbreak of shigellosis infected more than 7,000 people in North Carolina. Natural outbreak? Terrorist attack? Government test?

Highly infectious, shigellosis is highly transmissible in food, water and from person to person by fecal matter contaminated hands – personal hygiene is essential to prevent passing on or getting the infection.

In September, October and November of 2001 more than 2,000 cases of *Shigella dysenteriae* dysentery were diagnosed in school children in Cincinnati, Ohio. Shigellosis is almost never fatal, and only a few Cincinnati cases required hospitalization. Antibiotics generally cure individual infections and in the absence of drugs the disease will run its course of fever, stomachaches and bloody diarrhea in a few weeks. Natural outbreak? Terrorist attack? Government test?

Escherechia coli bacteria has been sprayed on salad bars by individuals but alert customers foiled the attempt to infect people – the most virulent strain of *E. coli* is 0157:H7 and can under certain circumstances cause death.

Warnings, alerts and General Recognition of an attack:

The Office of Homeland Security of the U.S. government has created a five category color-coded warning and alert system similar to the military Defcon (Defense Readiness Conditions) system. The purpose of the system being to give the domestic security agencies (i.e.- local police, state police, Secret Service, FBI, etc.) and the general public some sense of the degree of a threat and to some degree what preparations to make:

- Red – severe risk: close public and government buildings; monitor or close airports and major sporting events; increase or redirect emergency personnel.

- Orange – high risk: coordinate security with armed forces; restrict access to threatened sites; take additional precautions for public safety.

- Yellow – significant elevated terrorist risk: increase surveillance of critical locations; implement contingency emergency plans.

- Blue – general or guarded threat: review emergency response procedures; give public information.

- Green – low risk: check facilities for vulnerability to terrorist attack; train personnel.

Protection of individuals and large populations from chemical and biological warfare covers a wide range of approaches. First of all, a chemical or biological attack is not always immediately recognized because the agents are often colorless, odorless and tasteless. Be alert to "quiet" attacks, indicators include:

- Oily or dust aerosol drops on outside surfaces.
- Dead or dying insects, birds, fish or mammalian pets or wildlife.
- Unexpected sprays, gasses or aerosols.
- Unusual odors (i.e.- almonds, apricot pits, newly cut hay or grass).
- Unauthorized spraying in your area.
- Human victims showing symptoms of nausea, respiratory distress, convulsions, disorientation.
- Low lying "clouds or fog" not predicted by weather forecast or season; clouds of dust or colored particulate substances.

What to do in case of an attack:

- Be ever alert for weather or attack warning signs or sirens. Early detection of and recognition of an attack enhances your survival potential.
- Move upwind from source of attack.
- If evacuation is impossible move indoors and climb to highest floor (many biological and chemical agents are heavier than air).
- Close all windows, exterior doors, chimney dampers and heating and cooling systems.
- Cover mouth and nose with mask, cloth soaked in water and baking soda; cover head, arms and legs.
- If splashed with an agent, immediately wash it off with copious amounts of warm soapy water.
- Letters containing chemical or biological agents should be handled as little as possible. If there was a "puff" of dust or particles from the envelope notify authorities when they arrive. Place such envelopes in a sealed plastic food bag. Vigorously wash hands, face and hair before calling for help.
- In a car, shut off outside air intake vents and close windows if gas has not contaminated the interior.
- Seek medical help as soon as possible even if symptoms have not appeared.

Preparing a "safe-haven" or "Panic room":

In some instances an entire neighborhood or city (i.e.- Mina Mata, Japan; Bhopal, India) can be affected by an industrial accident or by chemical warfare agents. If your location makes this a possibility it is wise to establish a sealed chemical/biological safe-haven in your home:

- Select an inner room on an upstairs floor with the least number of windows.
- Choose a large room with access to a bathroom and telephone.
- Avoid rooms with window or wall mounted air conditioners as they are tough to seal.
- Close all windows, doors and shutters.
- Seal all cracks around window and doorframes with wide very sticky electrical or duct tape.
- Cover windows and exterior doors with 6-mil. plastic and seal with duct tape.
- Seal all openings including keyholes with wet rags and duct tape.
- Shut down all window and central air and heating units.
- Stockpile protective clothing including masks, rain suits, boots and rubber gloves.
- Keep a three-day supply of water and "no cooking necessary" food.
- Store weapons, flashlights, portable radios, batteries, first aid kit, bottle and can openers, knife, tools (electrical, carpentry, axe, bolt cutters, scissors, fire extinguishers, etc.), extra set of vehicle keys, money, prescription glasses, baby supplies, prescription meds, antibiotics, picture identification papers and extra blankets.

There are four steps to a Red Cross family safety program:

- Ask local officials for most likely disasters (i.e. – floods, tornadoes, hurricanes, earthquakes, etc.) – get information on how to prepare for each. Learn your communities warning signals, watch the TV news before you go to bed each night. Find out how to help the elderly, disabled and pets. Find out about disaster preparedness at your workplace, schools and daycare.

• Meet with your family and discuss why and how you need to prepare for a disaster. Pick two places to meet. – just outside your house in case of fire or outside your neighborhood if you can't return home because of blocked access. Ask an out of state friend or relative to be a family contact – everyone must known this number. Know what to do in case of an ordered evacuation or declaration of marshal law.

• Post emergency phone numbers on a home bulletin board, office and in each family members phone book. Teach children how and when to dial 911. Show family members how to turn off valves and switches for water, gas and electricity. Maintain adequate insurance coverage. Show each family member where the fire extinguishers are and how to use them. Install smoke detectors on each level of your home near or in the bedrooms. Conduct home hazard hunt. Take a Red Cross or Boy Scout CPR and first aid course. Find best escape routes from house including rope ladders from second floor.

• Practice, update and maintain your plan. Have a drill every six months. Use and replace stored water every three months and stored food every six months. Test and recharge batteries, fire extinguishers and smoke detectors monthly.

Personal preparation for environmental, biological and chemical agent disasters:

1) Well nourished individuals with a high level of natural or artificial (vaccinations) immunity and good post attack support are more likely to survive; unprotected infants, the infirm, the undernourished and seniors are more likely to succumb – therefore the daily supplementation with all 90 essen-

tial nutrients, the use of immune system stimulating herbs (Echinacea, noni juice, green tea, killer bee propolis, olive leaf, grape seed, garlic, onion, cayenne, etc.) and cholostrum antibodies are imperative practices for maximum individual pre-exposure protection.

2) In a war-footing environment with the risk of biological warfare vaccinations for smallpox, anthrax, plague and the use of antiviral and antibacterial herbs (garlic, cayenne, olive leaf, ginger root, etc.) and cholostrum antibodies should be used as a pre-emptive protection program.

3) The twice or three times daily use of a good antibacterial/antiviral hand and body soap on the scalp, face, neck, arms and hands will leave a low level of germicidal residue which can help reduce the risk of damage and death from biological infectious agents.

4) A supply of a good liquid laundry detergent and a small refillable garden sprayer should be kept in the vehicle, kitchen, bathroom, bed room, garage, workplace along with 20 gallons of water per person for flushing and washing the face, eyes and body to decontaminate and rid ones skin of contact sources of bacteria, virus and chemicals including dust, smoke and sticky gels.

5) Dust masks (N95 or N100)*, respirators and gas masks, rain suits, ponchos, rubber boots, plastic or rubber gloves can offer some limited protection against microbe and chemical laden dust, smoke, aerosols, sprays – remember, chemicals and microbes on protective clothes are still dangerous! Protective garments must be washed (decontaminated) with detergents and flushed away before one can enter a clean area and the clothing can safely be removed!

6) Antibiotics include ciprofloxacin (500 mg b.i.d. for 60 days), doxycycline (100 mg b.i.d. for 60 days) and penicillin (500 mg t.i.d. for 60 days) for anthrax and tularemia; streptomycin, gentamicin, tetracyclines and fluoroquinolones for plague can be used after exposure - syrups of these antibiotics

should be on hand for use in small children, pre-emptive use of vaccinations for smallpox and anthrax, antitoxin for botulism should be considered.

7) Atropine and atropine containing herbs are effective in countering the effects of nerve gases such as sarin, tabun and VX – full protection and recovery is possible if immediate action is taken.

8) Water requirements per person include two quarts of drinking water; hot environments can double this need; children, nursing mothers and the infirm can require even more. Store two weeks of water per person. Never ration water – find more tomorrow! If you need to find water outside the home use rainwater, water from moving water (streams, rivers), ponds and lakes. Do not drink floodwater! Let outside water set for 24 hours to allow large particulates to settle out; then pour the outside water through a cloth that has been soaked in diluted bleach water to filter out sediment, floating matter and glass. You can sterilize outside water with common household liquid chlorine bleach that contains 5.25 percent sodium hypochlorite. Add 16 drops of the bleach to each gallon of water and let stand a minimum of 15 minutes – better yet overnight. You can boil water for five minutes but this procedure requires the use of fuel and fire. Hidden water in the home can include water from the hot water heater (turn off electricity or gas), pipes, ice cubes and the reservoir or water closet from the toilet.

9) Have a two-week supply of food for each person in the house. Keep even canned, boxed and bottled food in dry, dark cool places. Keep food covered at all times. Close boxes and containers tightly after each use. Wrap cookies, crackers, dried fruit and nuts in re-sealable food bags and put them into larger cans or bottles with tight lids to avoid attracting pests. Inspect all food for spoilage before use. Date and cycle all food supplies. Eat at least one well-balanced meal each day. Consume enough calories to do work and function properly.

Include all 90 essential nutrients and a protein drink in each day's food program. Have a complete sweat replacement drink concentrate to fortify water when sweating occurs. Unlike water, food can be rationed if necessary except for kids and pregnant women. Don't stock salty food or soft drinks as they increase thirst and can cause dehydration. If the electricity goes off use perishable food from the fridge first, then food from the freezer and lastly the non-perishable food.

* Dust masks recommended by the CDC have a minimum rating of N95, meaning it screens out 95% of particles down to about a 0.3 micron particle size. Mask rated N100 screen out up to 99.97% of such particles. Infectious disease experts say the thinner generic paper masks often worn by hospital personnel would not be effective against anthrax.

Experts agree that the United States government and hospitals are not prepared to deal with large - scale biological or chemical attacks of any scope on the American public and that individuals who will survive are the ones who take personal responsibility and are maximally prepared in advance for any event.

It seems to us that seniors and grandparents are the ones who have the patience, cool heads, experience, wisdom and time to be the family and neighborhood designates for monitoring and delegating these responsibilities.

Additional reading:

Wallach, J.D. and Lan, Ma: Let's Play Doctor. Wellness Publications. Bonita, California. 1989.

Wallach, J.D. and Lan, Ma: Let's Play Herbal Doctor. Wellness Publications. Bonita, California. 2001.

Wallach, J.D. and Lan, Ma: RARE EARTHS: forbidden cures. Wellness Publications. Bonita, California. 1994.

Wallach, J.D. and Lan, Ma: Dead Doctors Don't Lie. Heritage Publications. Nashville, Tennessee. 2000.

Cole, L.A.: The Eleventh Plague: The Politics of Biological and Chemical Warfare. W.H. Freeman. New York. 1997.

Drell, S.D. et al (ed.): The New Terror: Facing the Threat of Biological and Chemical Weapons. Hoover Institution Press. Stanford, California. 1999.

Falkenrath, R.A. et al: America's Achelles' Heel: Nuclear, Biological, and Chemical Terrorism and Covert Attack. MIT Press. Cambridge, Mass. 1998.

Lederberg, J. (ed): Biological Weapons: Limiting the threat. MIT Press. Cambridge, Mass. 1999.

Miller, J. et al: GERMS. Simon & Schuster. New York, NY. 2001.

Osterholm, M.T. and Schwartz, J.: Living Terrors: What America Needs to Know to Survive the Bioterrorist Catastrophe. Delacorte Press. New York, NY. 2000.

Chapter 13

Financial security for centenarians

*"I would rather be paid for one percent of the efforts
of a hundred people than for 100 percent of my own."*

—John Paul Getty
First American Billionaire

Workers who were born after 1960 aren't eligible for full Social Security benefits until they're 67 years of age. Eligibility phases in for workers born between 1938 and 1959. You can start taking benefits as early as age 62, but your benefits will be reduced by as much as 30%, depending on when you were born!

Nine out of 10 senior Americans 65 years of age or older receive Social Security benefits. Sixty three percent of American seniors depend on their benefits for 50% of their income. For 30% of seniors, Social Security is 90% or more of their annual income. Eighteen percent of senior Americans rely on Social Security for 100% of their annual income.

By taking benefits while you're still working can be costly. In 2002, workers ages 62 to 64 can earn up to $11,280 with no reduction in Social Security benefits. But if you earn more than that, $1 in Social Security benefits will be withheld for every $2 you earn over $11,280. "It's like a 50% tax on your benefits," says AARP!

If you retire at age 62 and had been making $70,000 per year, you will earn $1,293 in monthly Social Security benefits. If you wait until eight months after your 65th birthday you'll get $1,717 a month. If you wait until your 70th birthday, you'll receive $2,328 per month. You don't get any extra benefit for waiting to apply for Social Security until after age 70. You can estimate your specific benefits by going to Social Security's Web site: www.ssa.gov.

Deciding when to apply for Social Security benefits would be easy if we all knew when we are going to die. Most of us aren't privy to our death date, however, if you're in poor health you might want to start collecting your benefits. If you're healthy and your family is comprised mostly of 80 and 90 year olds then you might want to delay applying for your benefits – if you plan on living past 74, you'll be better off to wait until you're 70 to apply for benefits.

Your Social Security check should be your monthly disposable income to have fun-time with, not your sole source of monthly income!

The current American retirement statistics are abysmal: 1% of American retirees at age 65 are "well off" with an annual retirement income of $50,000 or more after 40 years of work; 4% are "comfortable" with less than $50,000 annual income; and 95% live in constricted, fixed income lifestyles in or near the poverty level of $25,000 per year.

Another way to look at the financial future of the retiree is that out of every hundred Americans entering the workforce at age 18 by age 65 years 20 will have died, 39 live in poverty, 24 are barely surviving on subsistence level incomes, 14 can support themselves and 3 have annual incomes of over $50,000.

The average American works for three to ten different companies over their productive life, few understand the 401(k) benefit and as a result don't accumulate a full retirement program in any single job. A very few do work for a single company for 20 to 30 years; however, a single source of retirement income is not a guarantee for an endless flow of money – ask former

Montgomery Ward, Bethlehem Steel and Enron employees or investors.

A successful financial life as a 100 year old dictates that one not listen to the financial advice of 99 percent of the people they know who will statistically wind up broke at retirement. Robert Kiyosaki, the "best-selling author" of Rich Dad Poor Dad, points out that the traditional concept of a good job and benefits being the answer to a safe financial retirement will almost always fall far short of producing the desired retirement.

Rather, most retirees are forced to sell their home, their major "investment" that they worked and slaved for over 30 years because they had refinanced it and the house had then become a liability – a monthly cash sink.

In November of 2001 Alcoa aluminum laid off 6,500 employees and closed six plants because of high wages and benefits; Bethlehem Steel filed for bankruptcy because they couldn't continue paying the monthly retirement benefits to 73,000 retirees; Verizon cut 29,000 employees in 2001 and an additional 10,000 employees in 2002; early in January of 2002 Enron, the Houston based energy giant, accumulated $80 billion in debt and became the largest bankruptcy in U.S. history and vaporized billions of dollars of retirement programs for tens of thousands of ex-employees and mutual fund investors; late in January of 2002 K Mart, the second largest retail outlet in the U.S. filed for bankruptcy – the post WTC attack stock market free fall caused many benefit and retirement funds to severely contract or dry up altogether.

In 2001 numerous business icons went under leaving retirees penniless. Through mid-November 2001 more than 219 publicly traded companies had declared bankruptcy, far surpassing the 176 that filed during all of 2000. American goods production dropped for 13 months in a row in and 3.8 million workers were laid off in 2001 – the post World Trade Center attack financial down slide was the worst since the Great Depression.

Who would have thought that Montgomery Wards at 125

years of age would declare bankruptcy – after all they created Rudolph the red nosed reindeer and the money back guarantee! Enron? Bethlehem steel? Kaiser Aluminum? Polaroid? Global Crossing? K-Mart? Converse shoes! Swissair? Alamo car rental!

In January 2002 Ford fired 35,000 employees, 22,000 in the U.S. and Canada, closed five assembly plants and ended production of four cars including one of their luxury flagships, the Lincoln Continental; in February 2002 Goodyear laid off 35,000 employees; in March of 2002 K-Mart closed 280 stores in 20 states and terminated 22,000 employees; in April 2002 Arthur Anderson laid off 7,000 employees.

The average American senior-to-be believes that investments (i.e.- real estate, gold, stocks, mutual funds, 401(k), IRAs, annuities, insurance programs, etc.) are the bulwark of financial and health security to the retiree – yet according to the U.S. Department of Labor only one percent of retirees fixated on traditional investments retires well off with over $50,000 of annual income, four percent retires to what is generally considered a "comfortable" life and 95 percent of Americans retire at the poverty level with an annual income below $25,000.

"Retirement home":

Government and insurance support for nursing home care is only 60% of actual costs. If you pay for the balance of the costs of nursing home care you might get a tax deduction but there is no chance of any cash flow to you.

No one looks forward to living in a nursing home as they get older because of the horror stories of neglect and abuse and as a result the number of people enrolling in nursing homes is down 10% in 2001 compared with previous years.

In our experience, the best way to deal with senior housing for a family member is to buy a small two-bedroom two-bathroom house or a duplex instead of paying for a nursing home unit or bed, plus you get the tax benefits of income property – Robert

Kiyosaki describes rental property as zero tax money.

If special medical care is needed for a senior living at home, then obtain the services of a visiting nurse or home care aide. The cost of a visiting home care aide can be 30% to 50% less than nursing home care in a shared room – an additional benefit is you don't have to deal with a medical doctor, you are their boss and get to tell them to give mom and dad their vitamins and minerals! When the time comes and grandma goes to heaven at age 120 years, the house or duplex can be rented out as a source of passive income or sold and the investment recouped.

Good health benefits myth:

The average person falsely believes that their company health benefits will cover all future health needs. Because of this false belief many employees will often take lesser salary levels for a job with the promise of a "good medical benefit" package.

Rising health care costs will always outstrip private and government insurance benefits. The elderly and disabled users of Medicare HMOs used 50% more of their own finances for medical care in 2001 than they did three years earlier.

Personal spending for health care rose 43% between 1999 and 2001 for an out of pocket cost of $1,195 for those in good health and 63% increase in 2001 to an out of pocket cost of $3,578 for those Americans in bad health! Increases are expected to be even steeper in future years.

The paycheck benefit myth:

The big financial problem in retirement is a lack of a consistent liquid monthly cash flow – when you need cash your real estate investment may have dropped in value and you can't sell or rent it out – an investment that you're making payments on that does not produce positive monthly income has become a liability; it might be six months or more, before your bonds or CDs mature

– if you have this problem you are missing a big piece out of your retirement financial program.

The successful retirees learn early that the concept of depending on a paycheck (earned income) and employee benefits alone for a joyous, quality and pain free retirement is a huge problem at retirement because of the wants people have during their productive years. Large burdens of personal, credit card and bank loan debt are incurred because people who have paychecks have good credit. Good credit is soon followed by the acquisition of the big house, the time-share, the big car, the big boat, country club dues, the RV, the snow mobile and other toys all of which are bought on credit.

Any negative financial change (layoff, no overtime, rise in healthcare costs, rise in gasoline prices, rise in electricity prices, stock market downturn, kids getting older, college, new car purchase) results in a financial crisis; savings have to be cannibalized to make the payments on the mortgage, time shares and loans; savings are depleted; the bank takes back the toys; personal credit rating is lost – game over.

The successful retiree builds multiple sources of passive cash flow that are truly passive income early in life (although it is never too late). Passive income is income that flows to you requiring little or no effort once it is established. Ideally passive income sources negate the necessity for a paycheck and will pay for the luxuries so that your paycheck budget will be more than sufficient to cover your daily expenses.

If your paycheck goes away then your passive income should be large enough to cover your mortgage payments and your bills – if not, then you need more passive income. It takes a very highly motivated person to build additional passive income sources when everything seems to be "going well." The average person interprets lots of available overtime as things "going well." The average person then will overbuy toys and other liabilities on time payments – when the overtime stops or is reduced significantly a financial crisis occurs; the music stops and you are left without a chair!

The "more education" trap:

In 1978 as a widower with "four hungry children and a crop in the field" as Kenny Rogers sings, I knew I needed passive income, preferably multiple sources of passive income – I was motivated!

I thought I needed more education to gain more passive income; so, being the perennial student I did the natural thing, I went back to school without a second thought. I just needed to learn how to make a passive income. I needed to diversify. I needed more education!

I had already worked on my agricultural and veterinary degrees at the same time, so it didn't seem too outrageous to get business education at the same time I was a medical student. While an ND medical student, I studied part time outside of and in addition to my medical school work and got an insurance license and sold insurance; I thought of buying a McDonalds restaurant and took their management course – but it turned out that they were too time intensive, they were not the passive sources of income that I was looking for. Initially it seemed like my efforts to learn the insurance and fast food businesses was a dead end and a waste of time.

I got more education and gained in business skills that I had previously known little or nothing about, but the insurance business required significant amounts of time invested in cold contacting (a great skill) and burning a lot of shoe leather to build a residual income; the hamburger business required standing behind a counter 12 hours a day or supervising a manager who would be paid out of the gross profits – both took me in the wrong direction, they gave me less time with my family, employees to be concerned about and took time away from my medical studies.

I had learned a lot of basic skills in sales, employee training and motivation and inventory management in the insurance and fast food businesses but I gave up on them as being the source of true residual income that was going to set me free.

Rental property and apartments:

Rental property can be a double-edged sword. The main requirement of successfully owning rental property as a source of passive income is that it must generate a positive cash flow – if you have to pay the mortgage and maintenance of the unit out of your household budget you have only acquired a very dangerous financial liability that could cause you to enter a new chapter in your life – Chapter 7 bankruptcy!

Location is everything. If one acquires rental property near a college, university, hospital, transportation crossroads or large factory the odds are, if it is well maintained, your rental property will have a high occupancy rate. If your property is isolated way out in the cornfield and inconvenient, they might not come!

Rental property can be used to provide economical housing for a loved one as an alternative to a nursing home.

There are rental units that are designed to be basic dwellings for singles, couples or families and there are units that are designed for commercial use by businesses or professional offices. In good economic times both are good investments, in tight economic times long-term business leases are the best bet.

People often forget that rental real estate is a liability as long as they are making the mortgage payments out of their pocket without any rental or lease fees coming back to them. In a soft economic market it might be years before you can find a suitable renter and there goes your cash reserves that you accumulated over many years.

Passive cash flow from another non real estate source should be in place to cover real estate mortgages if renters and leases are not forthcoming in a soft economy. Back up systems are absolutely essential for a successful retirement at any age but especially when you are 100 years old.

An innovative way to harness the power of network marketing to acquire rental property is to "sponsor" the corporation or LLC (limited liability corporation) that owns the property into your network marketing down-line as a distributor, then sign up new distributors under the corporation to build a financially viable down-line.

The corporation can legitimately qualify and be eligible for commission checks by purchasing soaps, detergents, cleansers and landscaping materials for use on the property. Commission income can be used to upgrade the property, market the property and contribute towards the mortgage payments. What a concept, use passive income to acquire passive cash flow assets!

Robert Kiyosaki, "best-selling" author of *Rich Dad, Poor Dad*, and noted lecturer on financial success suggests acquiring two positive cash flow multiple dwellings each year.

Stock investment:

A diverse stock portfolio can be a valued source of passive income. My daddy always said, "Don't invest in the stock market if you need access to the money in the next five years." The advice says, "Generate disposable passive money that you don't need for basic expenses to invest in the stock market rather than taking money from your paycheck and monthly household budget."

The first maxim of managing a stock investment is that "there is no such thing as a risk-free investment." The avoidance of one type of investment risk is to take on another type of risk or loss. The safest investments give the lowest returns and the biggest potential winners offer the greatest potential for loss. NEVER PUT EVERYTHING AT RISK!

The really big winners in the stock market are the individuals who buy a stock before it is a well known icon – buy a stock when it is worth $1 and sell some or all of it when it reaches $80 – don't buy stock at its peak when it reaches $80 and everybody is excited as it is then too late for that opportunity!

The safest and easiest plan for financial survival and stability, as a centenarian, is to diversify ones sources of investment income and passive income like successful corporations. Ten sources of diversified residual income, including rental property, network marketing commissions, stocks and bonds, are better than one or two – your Social Security check should be disposable income to have fun with, not your sole source of income at the age of 100!

Mutual funds:

Some basic rules for IRA or 401(k) investments (employer stock should be less than 5% of your 401(k) stock package – any more than this is very risky, i.e. – Enron, Global Crossing, Nortel, Providian Financial) and withdrawals after retirement at 65 will increase the probability that they will provide ongoing income after the age of 100.

Preferably you need to withdraw taxable accounts first because you're paying taxes on dividends and interest from your taxable accounts, bonds, long-term bonds, and cash, including fund accounts. Then next withdraw from tax-friendly individual stocks and mutual funds. Because of the tax benefits, delay opening IRAs until you really, really need them; the last asset to be tapped should be the Roth IRAs because they are in effect tax havens.

A common mistake at retirement is to withdraw monthly draws from your retirement funds at or just below what they are earning – earning 12% withdraw 10% is a common pattern.
Experts show that if you withdraw 7% of an all-stock portfolio the first year and increase the withdrawal by 3% each year to hedge inflation you have less than a 38% probability of your funds lasting 25 years! Conversely you have a 70% chance of your retirement funds lasting 25 years if you initially withdraw 5% and add 3% annually for inflation.

With a retirement fund that consists of 80% stocks and 20% bonds you can withdraw 5% and expect it to have a 79% probability of the cash flow lasting 25 years – drop your withdrawal to 4% and you have a 95% chance of the fund lasting 25 years.

When you have other sources of passive income such as rental property income and network marketing income, then a modest withdrawal of only 4% from your stock portfolio will be sufficient, and will not constrict your life style.

New IRA rules can benefit your heirs by "stretching" tax deferral beyond your death. To safely plan for a "stretch" IRA, you will need good planning while you're still alive and good follow-up by your heirs after you die. DO NOT LEAVE 401(k) ACCOUNTS BEHIND WHEN YOU LEAVE A JOB! Roll them over into your IRA. Don't name your estate as a beneficiary – it would vaporize the IRA accounts tax status.

The greatest risks in mutual fund investing includes:

- Market risk. This is the BIG RISK a.k.a. the principal risk – it's the risk that an economic downturn vaporizes your money (i.e. – Enron).
- Purchasing power risk. Often times called the inflation risk – this is the risk of avoiding risk – it is at the opposite end of the scale from market risk. If you are too conservative your money can't grow fast enough to keep up with inflation (i.e. – savings account or in a mattress).
- Interest-rate risk. This is where one faces income declines when a bond or CD matures and you need to reinvest your funds. Bumping up returns using higher yielding, longer term securities, creates the potential of getting bogged down in inflation if the rates change in the short term.
- Shortfall risk. You can end up with shortfall risk by being too conservative or too aggressive.
- Timing risk. The probabilities of mutual stocks making money over the next 20 years is very good, the probability of mutual funds making money over the next 20 months is low (don't invest in stock if you need the money soon).
- Liquidity risk. A risk affected by current market pressures, it affects everything from junk bonds to foreign stocks.

- Opportunity risk. This is the greed factor kicking in – "jump in now or you will miss out." Opportunity risk works just the opposite of "rational" human thought – people see "opportunity" at the worst time when markets peak (worst time to buy) and fret at having to buy when stock values are low (best time to buy).
- Political risk. Government actions out of your control affect your stock values (Clinton shutting down military bases that resulted in 2001 – 2002 recession).
- Societal risk. This is "world event" risk – example, stocks dropped dramatically after World Trade Center and anthrax attacks.
- Additional risk includes currency risk, credit risk, etc.

Home based business:

Owning ones own home-based business that produces a residual cash flow is an absolutely necessary part of any successful retirement financial program – it is the only true hedge against inflation and recession. You can have the lifestyle of a millionaire if you have a residual passive positive cash flow of $5,000 to $10,000 per month over and above your paycheck and the ability to increase this amount without significant additional effort, overhead or employees.

A second benefit of owning your own business is that you get to legally take advantage of the tax laws designed to encourage the growth of small business. There are no tax benefits for employees except having additional children. There are no tax benefits for new college or high school graduates except for owning their own business – when there is an economic downturn and jobs are hard to come by, more new graduates will start their own businesses. The average American employee earns $25,000 per year while the average small business owner makes more than $50,000 per year.

You can sell your home-based business, will it to your survivors or you can continue to run it long after the 100-year old mark.

There are three basic types of home-based business' to consider:

Type 1 – **Start up** a business by the bootstraps – find a need and fill it, a do it yourself project. Many American millionaires start a multi-million dollar business in their garage.

The advantage of a bootstrap startup business is high profit and 100 percent control of the daily operation.

The downside is you are responsible for all aspects of the daily operation (i.e.- labor, personnel, payroll, travel, accounting, research, production, marketing, collections, utilities, etc.).

Type 2 – Purchase a **franchise**. The benefit of buying a national franchise is you purchase a turnkey operation and a perfected operating and marketing system, success is almost 100% assured. The associated corporate training, marketing and advertising systems are all tried, true and guaranteed.

The downside of purchasing a franchise is an airtight restrictive contract and a large initial franchise fee, employees and a significant time investment.

Type 3 – Join a reputable **network marketing** company. Donald Trump is famous for saying during a TV interview, "If I lost it all I would build a network marketing business." The benefits of joining an established network marketing company include low startup cost (as low as $6), they have established consumable products and the parent company calculates and pays out the commissions. You work out of your house and as a result you have low overhead, high profit, tax benefits and you control your time and can develop large residual incomes. Started early enough, it's not too outrageous to build network marketing passive incomes that exceed six-figure annual incomes.

In 1980, two years before graduating medical school, a young woman invited me to a business training meeting; she had learned of my personal situation and that I was looking for passive income and she said, "I think you will be very interested in this truly passive income business." She introduced me to a network marketing presentation - a concept I had never heard of. I must have been a terrible prospect, I was 40 years old and no one had taken the trouble to introduce network marketing to me.

The young lady became my sponsor and began the process of teaching me the concepts and details of the network marketing compensation plan. It was in fact a passive income plan - I would earn money on the sales generated by members in my marketing group many of whom lived at great distances from me and I would never meet. The more people in my group and the better trainer I was the larger my check would be. What a concept!

In my personal view network marketing was a far more plausible concept for generating passive cash flow than insurance sales and owning a McDonalds franchise – the financial investment was small, overhead was not outrageous and the potential for cash flow and a six figure annual income was phenomenal. In fact in six months time I became a significant money earner ($5,000 per month) in network marketing with nutritional and personal care products.

In 1985 Ma Bell was broken up and "dial 1" was made available to all upstart long distance providers. To make a long story short I recognized the unique opportunity when MCI joined forces with the network marketing company I was involved with. They recruited the network marketing company's distributors to market their discounted long distance service. I got baby sitters for my kids, hired doctors to take care of my patients and cover my practice; I went to the largest truck stop in America and rented a motel room for a monthly rate of $400, installed a microwave and a small icebox and I was in business.

I signed up 3,000 over the road truckers in one month's time (I averaged 100 truckers signed up each day), most just wanted to save 50% on their $2,000 a month phone bill, but a few got the idea and signed up other truckers as they plied the American highways as distributors in my downline.

The bottom line was I established a serious passive income of tens of thousands of dollars that lasted for many years. I learned the value of passive income and how to take advantage of the unique opportunities lesson very well.

Dr. Ma Lan came into my life in 1987; we fell in love and were married on St. Valentine's Day in 1988 and became partners in life and partners in business. We started our own network marketing company, Wellness Lifestyles MLM, in 1989. The company's mission was to help people with their health and longevity. We wanted Americans to have an average life span of 100 years rather than 75 years. We knew it was already genetically possible for people to live to beyond 100 and we wanted to be the catalyst to make it happen for all Americans.

We were forced to co-join our little network marketing company into the larger network marketing company of our employer, which freed us from the daily task of doing the administration of our business, which allowed us to spend our time recruiting and training. After six years (and the Dead Doctors Don't Lie! audio tape) we had 85,000 people in our downline – we had figured it out!

Ma Lan and I learned the network marketing philosophy lesson well – help enough other people get what they want and you will always get what you want. By helping others earn passive income to improve and stabilize their lifestyle and retirement we could build a stable passive income to improve the lifestyle of our family – we could also use some of the passive income generated from our network marketing commission checks to purchase other forms of passive income such as apartment buildings, bed and breakfast facilities, hotels or health spas.

In short we could pay people and reward them to pass on the message of health and longevity through the power of network marketing rather than cannibalizing our other sources of income.

In 1997 with the help of our son Steve Wallach, Ma Lan and

I started American Longevity. American Longevity was built to incorporate everything good and valuable we had learned as network marketing distributors. We built a network marketing company that is more distributor-friendly than any other company and as a result we have a larger percentage of distributor success than any other network marketing company.

Robert Metcalfe, a founder of 3Com that brought the PalmPilot to the marketplace, developed an economic law for networks – "The economic power of a business is the square of the number of (active people) in the network." Ten people in your network marketing group gives your business the marketing power of 10 X 10 or 100 people!

A basic goal for your independent distributorship is to "duplicate." You can't do it all yourself otherwise your income is limited – remember Metcalf's Law. If you put on one home meeting per week you will only have the growth and sales power of four meetings per month. If you recruit and train ten people in your marketing group to put on one meeting per week each you will have the growth and sales power of 44 meetings per month. If you recruit and train 100 people in your group to put on one meeting per week you have the sales and marketing power of 404 meetings per month – that's netWORK marketing!

An innovative method of acquiring rental property using the power of network marketing is to sponsor the corporate entity that owns the property into your marketing group as a distributor. Sponsor other distributors under the property corporation to build a downline – qualify the property corporation by purchasing soaps, detergents and landscaping materials for use on the property. The commission check earned by the corporation can be used to upgrade the property, market the property and contribute towards the monthly mortgage payments.

The downside to network marketing is you need to be an organized self-starter – you are the boss (while you do have upline to mentor you; you don't have a time clock or a supervisor telling you what to do), you are the marketing department, you are the salesperson, you are the trainer, you are the recruiter and you are the customer service department.

We have heard a lot of people complain about their personal lack of success in network marketing. In our experience the only way to fail in network marketing is to do nothing! One's level of success in network marketing is directly proportional to ones efforts in network marketing. Remember, network marketing is not a lottery – its netWORK marketing!

Typically an individual's network marketing group takes two to five years to develop and mature if you are honestly working at it five to 10 hours each week – contrary to common belief, network marketing is not a get rich scheme. You will need to devote as much time educating yourself and building a successful network marketing business as you would for developing any other business – network marketing is a serious business not a lottery!

Tax benefits of a home based business:

Small business tax benefits change yearly so it's a good idea to have a good CPA to keep up with rule changes but there are basic principles to know and practice:

1) Always follow the letter of the law, make no attempt to cheat.

2) The cost of doing business is 100% tax-deductible.

3) Make a profit within 2 to 5 years of starting your business; a hobby doesn't count.

4) You get to deduct 50% of FICA by filing schedule C.

5) Keep good records; get your CPA to establish a system for you.

6) Education courses necessary for the operation of your business (i.e.- taxes, sales, motivation, marketing, computer, personnel, accounting, etc.) are 100% deductible no matter where they take place.

7) Document entertainment or promotional costs, including

home meetings, samples and motivational activities.

8) Employee functions are 100% deductible.

9) The limit for tax-deductible gifts to customers, clients, suppliers, employees and associates is $25.

10) The annual gift limit for kids is $10,000 each; gifted college funds are at a lower tax bracket.

11) Business meals are up to 50% deductible.

12) Dinner with spouse is deductible if there is a business purpose.

13) Deduct dues, fees, training, professional and business associations.

14) Deduct books, tapes, videos, manuals, etc.

15) Travel expenses are 100% deductible – keep good records.

16) Home office deduction (i.e.- % of mortgage, taxes, insurance, utilities, repairs, cleaning, depreciation, machines, computers, furniture, supplies, etc.).

17) Deduct health insurance at 100%

18) Lease business car deductions at 100%; business mile deductions for owned cars; beware of luxury limits on cars (promotion tool might be a better deduction).

19) Hire your spouse at a 100% deduction; there may not be employee tax on your spouses and kids paychecks in your state.

20) Save 30 – 40% of each commission check for quarterly tax payments and unforeseen business expenses (the GKW factor or God knows what) and unexpected investment opportunities (buy a duplex or an apartment building).

It is never too late to plan for your future – if you start after age 50 years of age you will just have to be more intense and go faster if you start late than if you had started earlier. The important thing for a successful retirement at age 100 is to have cash flowing to you! If you are paying mortgages on six rental properties out of your paycheck you are in trouble – they are a liability, not an asset if they are not paying their own freight or if another cash flow source is not covering the cost.

Dr. Ma Lan and I can envision 5 million American centenarians in the years 2050 beating the odds and living a well financed lifestyle of optimal health and longevity. It is all quite possible if you take action – don't forget, a paycheck, health and vacation benefits alone won't be enough when the time comes for retirement. The odds are not in your favor if you follow the standard 40-year plan – 95% of Americans retire at the poverty level below $25,000 per year!

Chapter 14

Dr. Wallach's See Food Diet

"At best, the RDAs are only a recommended allowance at antediluvian levels designed to prevent some terrible disease. At worst, they are based on conflicts of interest and self-serving views of certain positions of the food industry. Almost never are they provided at levels for optimum health and nutrition,"

—Senator Wm. Proxmire
Let's Live 1974

It is quite clear that what one eats and what one doesn't eat will directly affect ones health and longevity. The autopsies of more than 17,500 animals of 454 species and 3,000 humans revealed that every animal and every human that dies of "natural causes" dies of a nutritional deficiency disease. That's right, simple nutritional deficiency diseases cause most chronic degenerative diseases, illness and deaths in America!

Nutritional deficiency diseases are quite easily prevented and reversed with simple supplement programs in both animals and humans. While we Americans have spent more than $100 billion dollars in nutritional research for animals and designing diets that prevent and cure diseases in them, medical doctors continue to resist using nutrition to treat their human patients with nutritional formulas – there are no federal or state laws that require medical doctors to cure your disease even if a cure is known; there are no laws that require a medical doctor to prevent diseases in you even if a prevention is available.

We all would like to believe that doctors are doctors for altruistic reasons and they gain wealth because of their good works – however, statistics show that doctors follow the money. If they were to prevent diseases or cure all of their patients (which is quite easy) then they are soon out of business.

We know, for example, that even without supplementation of vitamins and minerals, the Mormons and Seventh Day Adventist gain up to ten years in additional longevity compared to the average American simply by giving up caffeine, alcohol and tobacco. Certain cultures (the Age Beaters) eat modest calorie diets that are rich in minerals and are blessed with a high average life span, Okinawa at 81.2, and a high percentage of centenarians; Russian Georgians boast 39/100,000 in centenarians.

Paying attention to percentages of carbohydrates, fat and protein can help control weight, add energy to your day and add fun to your day, however, "eating well" won't preclude the need for supplementation when it comes to living to be a centenarian – don't forget to supplement all 90 essential nutrients in optimal amounts daily.

Plants can't manufacture minerals and nutritional minerals do not occur in a uniform blanket around the crust of the earth – minerals occur in veins like gold and silver. Therefore, there are no guarantees that even by eating high quality foods, that a person can obtain all 90 essential nutrients without complete supplementation.

It quickly became apparent that the only hope for being universally successful in our goal to help the average American to surpass the current longevity average age of 75.5 and live to be over 100 was to employ the financially successful and results orientated methods used by the veterinary and agricultural industries preventive herd health programs.

No matter who they were, we wanted people to be able to see food and eat it without having to count calories, consider RDAs, become a food sociopath and "food combine" or to spend their lives shopping for special foods – so we decided to let people eat whatever they wanted – what a concept! See food and eat it! Dr.

Wallach's See Food Diet was born.

How to cook safely:

A general overview for safe cooking is, "If food makes noise or sizzles while cooking its too hot!" Poached or boiled foods only reach 212 F at sea level; baked and roasted foods reach 375 to 425 F; grilled foods reach 600 – 800 F; fried foods reach more than 800 – 1,200 F. Burnt animal fat of any kind turn into heterocyclic amines that can increase your risk of heart disease and breast, prostate and colon cancer by as much as 462%. Heated vegetable oils and margarines turn into trans fatty acids or free radicals, which increase your risk of cancer and heart disease.

We soft scramble eggs by slowly (without noise) melting a pat of butter in the skillet or sauce pan; the eggs are cracked and whipped with a whisk and poured into the skillet; use a rubber or fiber glass spatula to soft scramble the eggs – if you can play marbles with your scrambled eggs they have been over cooked!

Frying without shortening doesn't help prevent free radicals as most foods including eggs, red meat, fish, poultry and soy burgers have fat or oil within them that will turn into free radicals at elevated temperatures.

We cook red meat and poultry by salting the inside of a skillet and placing the meat or poultry on the salt – use tongs to turn rather than puncturing with a fork.

We grill a lot. I like to use a dry un-greased stainless steel cookie sheet on the grill to prevent flames from touching the food. I salt the surface of the cookie sheet to keep the food from sticking and to seal in the meats juices.

Steaming vegetables will fracture the phytate molecule found in raw vegetables (i.e.- carrots, broccoli, cauliflower, squash, etc.) making them safer to eat. Raw vegetables that snap when you break them contain phytates that form phytate/mineral complexes that are difficult to absorb.

Free radicals:

The first task was to focus our culinary effort towards eliminating the negative aspects of human eating habits without tampering with anyone's religious or conceptual choices of dietary needs or goals or their perception of just plain fun foods (i.e.-pizza, tacos, hot dogs, burgers – especially burgers – they're Dr. Wallach's favorite!!). So we decided first just to eliminate free radicals.

Free radicals come in many forms including margarine and cooking oils as trans fatty acids and burnt animal fats as heterocyclic amines.

To accomplish the universal elimination of free radicals we came up with a simple short list:

- No deep fried food (heated vegetable oils and burnt animal fats are killers)
- No vegetable oils (No! Not even extra virgin olive oil or frozen desserts)
- No vegetable oil containing salad dressing.
- No margarine (use butter, ghee or water for cooking)
- Do not eat burnt animal fat (heterocyclic amines increase cancer risk 462%).

It may take awhile to wean off of salad dressing so use Dr. Wallach's salad fork trick. Never put salad dressing on the salad, never dip salad into the salad dressing – dip your salad fork 1/4 inch into a side dish of dressing and eat small forks full of salad for taste without calories and free radicals. Colloidal mineral enriched noni juice makes a great "vinaigrette."

Contrary to popular belief **eggs** are good food. On the biological value scale for proteins (measures absorbability and usability), egg protein is 100 out of 100, they are the benchmark by which all other proteins are measured. Egg protein is especially good for growing kids and seniors. Low blood protein results in edema and swelling and loss of muscle mass – doctors want to give you diuretics to treat common edema when in reality what you need is to eat more eggs!

Salt:

Salt your food to taste. Doctors will tell you to restrict salt but remember, the Japanese consume 12 grams of salt per day and have 80% less cardiovascular disease than we do. Salt is the raw material to make stomach acid – without stomach acid you cannot efficiently absorb minerals, digest protein or absorb vitamin B12.

Salt does not cause high blood pressure and restricting salt will not reduce your risk of high blood pressure or add 10 seconds to your life – in fact restricting salt will shorten your life and make you very miserable.

Without stomach acid you are sure to develop bloating, burping, gastric reflux, G.E.R.D. (gastro esophageal reflux disease) and secondarily a wide variety of nutritional deficiency diseases for which doctors will want to treat you with drugs and surgery and put you at risk of injury and death – simply because you have a low stomach acid production or your stomach acid is being neutralized (i.e.- carbonated drinks, antacids, etc.).

Carbohydrates and Sugar:

The next step in Dr. Wallach's See Food Diet program is to seriously reduce or eliminate sugar, natural and processed (sugar loads increase the normal rate of mineral loss in sweat and urine by as much as 300% for 12 hours). There are no nutritional requirements for sugar or carbohydrate – you can make blood sugar, blood glucose and glycogen (animal starch) from fats and amino acids.

According to the U.S.D.A. Americans were eating ½ pound of sugar per person per year in 1895, and in the year 2002 Americans are eating 157 pounds of sugar per person per year – that's almost a half pound of sugar per day!

If you have honey on your English muffin for breakfast, ice cream for dessert at lunch and a pastry for dinner dessert no amount of mineral supplementation or no diet will ever allow you to keep up with or make up for your mineral losses.

Not only will you shed unwanted pounds by giving up sugar, your thinking will be clearer, you will be less irritable; you will have boundless energy (sugar consumption is the single biggest cause of fatigue) and if you have a history of hypoglycemia or hyperinsulinemia you will be half way home towards fixing your problem:

- no apple juice
- no grape juice
- no honey
- no molasses (cane juice, turbanado sugar, brown sugar)
- no table sugar
- no corn syrup
- no fructose
- no granola or energy bars
- no processed meats
- no BBQ sauce, no pasta sauce, no chili
- no candy
- no colas, non colas or other carbonated soft drinks
- no ice cream (exceptions include no sugar added ice cream), no sherbert
- no pastries
- no boxed or bagged cold or instant hot cereals

- no low fat yogurt or 98% fat free yogurt (it contains more sugar than regular yogurt).

If during the process of giving up sugar you get the "munchies" or feel the need to go on the classic "chocoholic" binge, take one ounce of plant derived colloidal minerals per 100 pounds of body weight – even if its ten times a day at the start (remember – cravings or pica are the sure sign of mineral deficiencies!!).

Carbonated drinks:

Give up carbonated drinks! Carbonated drinks neutralize stomach acid and you can't absorb minerals efficiently, digest protein or absorb vitamin B12 without stomach acid. Carbonated drink consumption increases the risk of many mineral deficiency diseases including osteoporosis (including fractures), arthritis, fibromyalgia, carpal tunnel syndrome, peripheral neuropathies, diabetes, hypertension, insomnia, obesity, etc.

Dietary fiber:

Reduce the consumption of high fiber meals to two per week. Whole grain bran, multi-grain breads and raw vegetables contain a substance called phytates. Phytates are carbon/phosphorus compounds that form phytate/mineral complexes that can't be absorbed efficiently leading to an increased risk of mineral deficiency diseases.

Caffeine:

Reduce caffeine consumption. Drink herbal teas rather than black ice tea and hot tea and decaffeinated coffee. Consuming 500 milligrams of caffeine per day will deplete mineral stores in the body.

Distilled water:

To ensure optimal health adult humans need to consume about eight to ten glasses of water each day – soft drinks, coffee and tea do not count as water because they have dehydrating properties.

Distilled water consumed as the sole source of drinking and cooking water can deplete mineral stores from your body. Adding one ounce of pure plant derived colloidal minerals per gallon of drinking or cooking water will counteract the "hungry water" effects of distilled water.

Supplement program:

Lastly, the unifying aspect of Dr. Wallach's See Food Diet is to supplement with all known essential nutrients to warranty your optimal daily intake of each – don't depend on food to be your major or sole source of micronutrients - remember plants can't manufacture minerals! Don't throw away significant numbers of healthful years like you would avoid junk mail. By faithfully sticking to a serious supplement program you will avoid a lot of unnecessary misery, save yourself a gob of money and add many, many healthful years to your life!

Table 12-1. The 60 Essential Elements, Metals and Minerals*

Aluminum	Gold	Rhenium
Arsenic	Hafnium	Rubidium
Barium	Holmium	Samarium
Beryllium	Hydrogen	Scandium
Boron	Iodine	Selenium
Bromine	Iron	Silica
Calcium	Lanthanum	Silver
Carbon	Lithium	Sodium
Cerium	Lutecium	Strontium
Cesium	Magnesium	Sulphur
Chloride	Manganese	Tantalum
Chromium	Molybdenum	Terbium
Cobalt	Neodymium	Thulium
Copper	Nickle	Tin
Dysprosium	Niobium	Titanium
Erbium	Nitrogen	Vanadium
Europium	Oxygen	Ytterbium
Gadolinium	Phosphorus	Yttrium
Gallium	Potassium	Zinc
Germanium	Praseodymium	Zirconium

* Many of the minerals on the list are not classically considered to be "essential", however, they all meet one or more of the criteria for an essential nutrient.

Table 12-2. Essential Vitamins for Human Health

Vitamin A
Vitamin B1 (Thiamine)
Vitamin B2 (Riboflavin)
Vitamin B3 (Niacin)
Vitamin B5 (Pantothenic acid)
Vitamin B6 (Pyridoxine)
Vitamin B12 (Cyanocobalamin)
Vitamin C
Vitamin D
Vitamin E
Vitamin K
Biotin
Choline
Flavinoids and bioflavinoids
Folic acid
Inositol

Table 12-3. The Essential Amino Acids

Valine
Lysine
Threonine
Leucine
Isoleucine
Tryptophane
Phenylalanine
Methionine
Histadine
Arginine*
Taurine*
Tyrosine*

* While not considered classic essential amino acids, their
deficiency does result in specific diseases.

Table 12-4. Essential Fatty Acids and Fats

Linoleic acid
Linolenic acid
Arachidonic acid*
Cholesterol*

*While not considered a classic essential fat, its deficiency does result in specific disease.

By employing Dr. Wallach's See Food Diet you can:

- be a member of any religion and supplement with the 90 essential nutrients.
- be a vegan and supplement with the 90 essential nutrients
- be a meat eater and supplement with the 90 essential nutrients.
- juice and supplement with the 90 essential nutrients.
- follow just about any dietary program you want if you supplement with the 90 essential nutrients.

To be sure there are certain adjustments you must make on a daily basis (i.e.- if you are going to eat a 72 ounce steak, you will need to take in additional supplemental calcium to avoid osteoporosis and arthritis; if you're a vegan you need to be aware of phytates and eat vegetables steamed instead of raw, take in your minerals between meals to maximize their absorption, double check B12 sources, etc.).

You can even "cheat" on Dr. Wallach's See Food Diet once or twice a month or special occasions (i.e.- holidays, birthdays, weddings, etc.) because your reserves of protective minerals will be filled to capacity and protect you from your occasional dietary sins!

Dr. Wallach's See Food Diet:

Breakfast suggestions include:

1) 2 poached eggs
   breakfast meat (i.e.- ground beef, steak, pork chop,
   salmon, trout, poultry)
   cheese
   tomatoes
   onions, peppers

2) 2 soft scrambled eggs, in butter, low temperature
   cottage cheese
   broccoli
   onions (baby pearl)
   ½ poppy seed bagel with1 pat real butter or Philadelphia
   cream cheese

3) whey protein/soy protein shake
   add raw or lightly poached egg
   add ½ cup chopped ice
   blend for 2 minutes

4) soft 2 egg vegetable omelette (tomato, slivered almonds,
   mushrooms, onions, bell pepper, broccoli, etc.)
   sliced tomatoes
   ½ poppy seed bagel with butter

5) grilled or poached salmon, trout or halibut (cover each fil-
   let with salted butter pats, chopped chives and dill or
   sweet basil)
   red onion slices
   sliced tomatoes
   one poached egg
   ½ onion bagel with butter or cream cheese

Lunch suggestions include:

1) large green leafy salads with carrots, celery, radishes
   and tomatoes, grilled chicken breast, beef steak or tuna
   steak, butter/sweet basil baste, whey "pudding" dessert

2) ½ roasted or grilled chicken
   mixed green salad, tomatoes, carrots, peppers, mushrooms, radishes, mineral enriched noni Goose Juice salad
   dressing (tastes like vinaigrette)

3) 6 – 8 oz burger (medium rare or rare)
   ½ bun (or better yet - no bun!)
   sliced onion
   sliced tomatoes
   sliced "stackers" dill pickle
   Swiss cheese
   Spicy mustard
   mixed green salad

4) grilled chicken breast sandwich (multi-grain bread)
   sliced tomatoes
   sliced onions
   spicy mustard
   cottage cheese

5) whey (sugar free) shake, add 2 oz ice cubes
   add a raw or lightly poached egg; blend for 1 minute

6) sardines (packed in mustard sauce, tomato sauce or water)
   sliced tomatoes
   artichoke hearts
   pimento stuffed green olives
   steamed carrot sticks

7) sardine stuffed peppers
    2 large bell peppers
    31/2 ounces sardines chopped
    1 cup steamed rice
    ½ - medium onion chopped
    1- cup tomato sauce
    1 beaten egg
    salt and pepper to taste
    fill pepper cavities with mix and bake at 350 degrees for
    20 minutes
    1 glass California white wine

8) vegetable beef or chicken soup (broccoli, onions, carrots,
    peas, tomatoes, string beans, celery, okra, etc.). Four
    ounces of grilled chicken (diced), ground or roast beef cut
    into cubes. Garlic salt to taste.

9) all beef bratwurst or hotdog without bun
    spicy mustard, chopped onions, chopped tomatoes, catsup
    sour kraut, beets
    6 ounces light beer

10) seven-bean soup (great laxative!) simmer for at least 2 – 4
    hours – continue to add water if needed.
    kidney beans
    pinto beans
    navy beans
    lima beans
    butter beans
    soy beans
    green beans
    pearl onions
    garlic salt to taste
    diced green tomatoes

Dinner suggestions include:

1) steak (6 – 10 ounce, 1 inch thick; medium rare), sprinkle
   with garlic salt
   large mixed Spring green salad, include onions, tomatoes,
   mushrooms, mineral enriched noni Goose Juice for salad
   dressing (tastes like vinaigrette)
   steamed vegetables
   one glass of red wine (merlot)
   2 scoops no sugar added ice cream

2) grilled or poached fish (salmon, trout, halibut, mahi-mahi,
   snapper) slivered almonds, chives, salted butter, dill,
   sweet basil or thyme
   steamed broccoli or carrots and peas or green beans
   vegetable soup or mushroom soup with clear broth
   one glass of white wine
   1 inch wedge of cheesecake

3) ½ roasted chicken, 1 Tblsp salted butter, sprinkle with ½
   tsp sweet basil
   large green salad, include onions, tomatoes, steamed
   carrots, celery, green peppers
   mixed steamed vegetables
   one sesame seed roll with butter
   one glass of white wine

4) 2 pork chops, 4 lamb chops or a lamb shank roasted medium or medium rare and juicy
   mixed steamed vegetables or asparagus
   large green salad, include wedges of lime
   herbal tea (peppermint)
   one glass of rose' or white wine

Salads and vegetables:

Steamed mixed vegetables

Broccoli
Broccoli, carrots, cauliflower
Green beans, slivered almonds, pearl onions
Peas, carrots (¼ inch cubes)
Peas, pearl onions
Mixed bell peppers (red, green, yellow, orange)
Beets, sliced onions
Okra, cooked tomato slices, pearl onions
Lima beans, pearl onions
Tomatoes, sliced onions

Salads

Romaine lettuce, shredded provolone cheese
Mixed spring greens (miner's lettuce, bib lettuce, dandelion leaves and flowers, etc.)
⅛ to ¼ head iceberg lettuce, tomato wedges, radishes, bell-pepper rings
Greek salad (feta cheese, salted olives, red onion rings), noni juice salad dressing.
Gouda or Brie cheese wedges, sliced tomatoes

Snacks and desserts:

* two ounces of salted mixed nuts

* whey/soy sugar free protein shakes or pudding

Key Lime Pie: mix one serving of Vanilla Nature's Whey according to directions. Add 2 Tblsp frozen limejuice; 1 graham cracker, 3 ice cubes.
Blend on high speed for 45 sec.

Egg Nog: Mix one serving of Vanilla Nature's Whey according to directions. Add ¼ tsp ground allspice, 1 lightly poached egg, 3 ice cubes. Blend on high speed for 45 sec.

Cinnamon Roll Supreme: Mix one serving of Vanilla Nature's Whey according to directions. Add ¼ tsp ground cinnamon, 1 tsp softened butter and 3 ice cubes. Blend on high speed for 45 sec.

Strawberry Cheesecake: Mix one serving of Vanilla Nature's Whey according to directions. Add 3 Tblsp of Jell-O's no-bake, reduced fat cheesecake mix, 3 low-fat vanilla wafers, 3 – 5 strawberries and 3 ice cubes. Blend on high speed for 45 seconds.

Chocolate Peanut Butter Cup: Mix one serving of Chocolate Nature's Whey according to directions. Add 1 heaping Tblsp of peanut butter and 3 ice cubes. Blend on high speed for 45 sec.

Double Deluxe Chocolate Fudge: Mix one serving of Chocolate Nature's Whey according to directions. Add 1 packet of sugar-free, fat-free hot cocoa mix and 3 ice cubes. Blend on high speed for 45 sec.

Cookies and Cream: Mix one serving of Chocolate Nature's Whey according to directions. Add 4 drops of peppermint extract and 3 ice cubes. Blend on high speed for 45 sec. Then add 4 low-fat chocolate wafers and blend at low speed for 10 sec.

Chocolate Mocha Mint: Mix one serving of Chocolate Nature's Whey according to directions. Add 1 and ½ heaping Tblsp of General Foods International Coffees Swiss Mocha sugar-free, fat-free instant coffee, 4 drops of peppermint extract and 3 ice cubes. Blend on high speed for 45 sec.

Banana Split: Mix one serving of Chocolate Nature's Whey according to directions. Add 1 banana, I oz. Osteo-fx, ⅛ cup chopped drained pineapple, 3-5 strawberries and 3 ice cubes. Blend on high speed for 45 sec.

* no sugar added ice cream or no sugar added yogurt (do not use fat free or low fat yogurt!)

* citrus fruit; one medium sliced apple

* carob, whey protein, rice flower "brownies" with walnuts

* sugar free cheese cake

INDEX

EPIGENETICS

The Death of the Genetics Theory of Disease Transmission.

EPIGENETICS Documents 10,000 years of medical superstition and mistakes, which includes: evil spirits, alchemy, magic, imbalance humors, stellar gods and witch craft, germs cause everything, the age of pharmaceuticals, and bad DNA trasmits all disease, the mapping of the genoma will allow doctors to cure all disease.

Up Coming

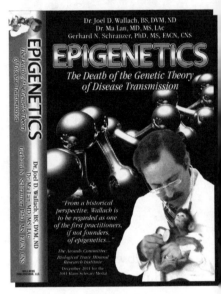

Finally the ultimate truth is discovered - "Through the proper use of nutrients the DNA script can perform at optimal levels to prevent and cure all none infectious diseases".

1-800-755-4656
www.drjwallach.com

Let's Play Doctor

The Book That "Orthodox" Doctors Couldn't Kill - "How to" maximize your genetic potential for health and longevity.

- Become your own primary health care provider
- Learn The Alternative Healing Arts
- Establish your own Health Clinic
- Establish a Home Pharmacy
- Home Surgery

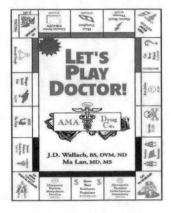

$14.95 - 10 or more $8.00 each

Rare Earths Forbidden Cures
Their Secrets of Health and Longevity

The definitive home reference on minerals, mineral deficiencies and their relationship to:

* Degenerative Diseases
* Learning Disabilities
* Criminal Behavior
* Birth Defects
* Addition
* Food Binges
* Depression
* Infertility and More!

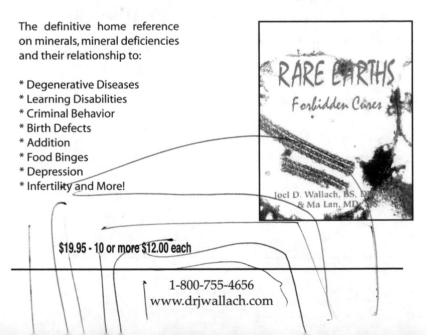

$19.95 - 10 or more $12.00 each

1-800-755-4656
www.drjwallach.com

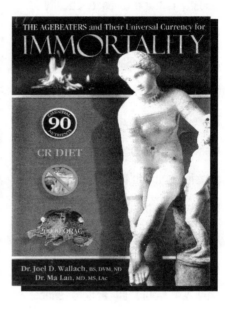

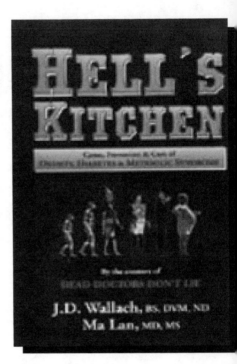

LET'S PLAY HERBAL DOCTOR

Learn about the pharmacologilcal
properties of plan herbs.
The history of herbal medicine
Learn how herbs work
Active constituents of
medicinal herbs
Growing, harvesting, selecting,
storage and processing of herbs

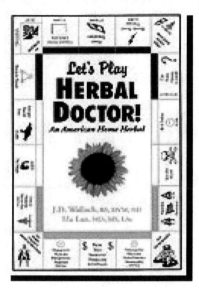

$19.95 - 10 or more $12.00 each

PASSPORT TO AROMATHERAPY

*Essential Oils Or "Essences" Are Highly
Concentrated Volatile Oils Extracted
From Aromatic Plants.*

Essential oils are legendary
for their anti-microbial
properties

Essential oils are legendary
for uplifting the emotions

$14.95 - 10 or more $8.00 each

**LEARN MORE ABOUT ESSENTIAL
OILS FROM THIS BOOK**

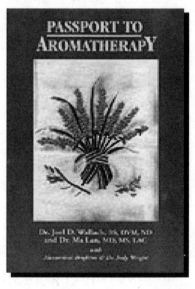

1-800-755-4656
www.drjwallach.com

BLACK GENE LIES

This book is a landmark expose that shows that the diseases

of the black population in

America, that the medical

community attributes to a

terrible "Black Gene", are in

fact caused by regional and

cultural eating habits and

nutritional deficiencies of trace

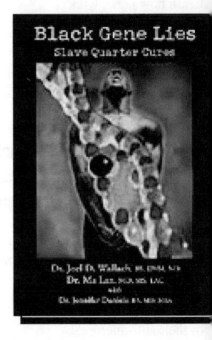

elements that are easily, safely and economically overcome

by the use of simple nutritional supplement programs and

herbal remedies

$19.95 - 10 or more $12.00 each

1-800-755-4656
www.drjwallach.com

GOD BLESS AMERICA!

- The epiphany
- American centenarians
- Medical dogmas/lies
- Health and longevity
- Weight loss
- Home defense and
- anti-terrorism plan
  Cash flow and tax plan
- Longevity recipes

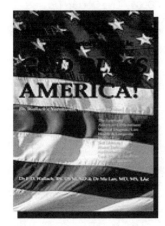

$14.95 - 10 or more $8.00 each

WALLach $Treet for kids

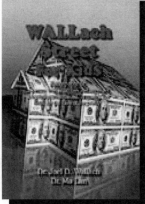

his book is about entrepreneurship, money and business
r the purpose of educating entrepreneurial kids, teens and
ung adults opportunities to find a "good jobs" in a chang-
g global economy, the obvious direction for entrepreneurs
to own their business. Ownership is the true measure of
wer of business

$19.95 - 10 or more $12.00 each

1-800-755-4656
www.drjwallach.com

Audio CDs

CD001	Dead Doctors Don't Lie	The origiinal tape that started it all
CD002	DDDL in Chinese, Korean,Spanish,Japanese	
CD003	Trust me, I am a Doctor	Dr.Wallach's 1996 health lecture series
CD004	Good Doctor, Bad Doctor	Dr.Wallach's 1997 health lecture series
CD005	Live Doctors Do Lie	
CD006	Medical Dogmas & Lies	Dr.Wallach's 2000 health lecture series
CD007	Medical Milking Machine	Dr.Wallach's 2000 health lecture series
CD008	What's Up Doc II	Health Products Information
CD009	Women,Athletes and Children	Menopause, ADHD and Athletes,2003
CD010	Medical Mouse Trap	Dr.Wallach's lecture on Doctor's continue edu
CD011	The Best of Dead Doctors Don't Lie	combination of DDDL I,II and III
CD012	Lucky Mo	Children's musical story
CD013	Hell's Kitchen	Dr.Wallach's 2004 health lecture series
CD014	God's Recipe	Health alternative to Ritalin
CD015	$10 Path to Financial Freedom	How to get your Youngevity products for free
CD016	Ferret Fat Pak 101	Weight loss product
CD017	Live Free or Die	Jonathan Emord
CD018	Healthier and Longer Life	
CD020	Dial MD for Murder	Dr.Wallach's 2004 health lecture series
CD030	Truth is Forever	Christian Songs by Dee Stocks
CD031	HE Has the Power to Heal	Christian Songs by Dee Stocks
CD033	WBA and Youngevity Opportunity	Dr.Wallach interviewed by Leroy MacMath -Atl physical and financial health
CD034	Black Gene Lies I	interviewed by Herbalist Dirk Twine - the top k diseases of African American
CD035	Black Gene Lies II	Dr.Wallach's lecture at World Changers Men's fellowship in Atlanta, GA
CD037	Tomato Warning	narration by Richard Dennis
CD046	Dead Athletes Don't Lie	
CD047	H5N1 Bird Flu	Dr.Ma Lan
CD048	Deadly Recipe	
CD056	Until Death Do Us Part	Outline information of Dr.Wallach's lectures
CD057	Energy Crisis	History on energy boost
CD058	Get your ACT together	Steve Wallach
CD059	New Best of DDDL	With 25 questions and answers
CD060	Tru Chocolate	Dr.Wallach , Sandy Elsberg and Elaine Lagatta
CD067	From Here To Immortality	Dr. Wallach
CD069	Aroma Therapy Oil	Dr. Wallach
CD070	Cerial Killer	Dr. Wallach
CD071	What Kills Billionaires	Dr.Wallach

**order 1-10: $3.00/each, 11-20: $2.00/each, 50 and more: $1.00/each
personalized CD label is available for minimum of 50 CD order.**

OTHER CDS

)028	Selenium	Dr.Gerhard Schrauzer
)028	Seeing is Believing	Dr.Pugh
)032	Quality,Quality	Richard Renton
)039	Beyond Juice	Ken Cole
)051	Foundation for Success	Richard Stocks
)052	Three Health Freedom Warriors	Dr.Wallach, Martin Luther King III, Jonathan Emord
)053	Juice Cures	Jay Kordich
)066	Who Made MD's King?	Dr. Peter Glidden
)068	Healing is Easy	Dr. Peter Glidden

PERSONALIZED CD

1) Minimum Order: 50/per title
2) Title: any title
3) Price: $1.00/per CD
4) Set-up fee: none

DVDs

		order 1-9 /	order 10
√D001	Let's Talk Minerals	$10.00	$7.00
√D002	Have You Heard	$10.00	$7.00
√D005	Is It Possible to Reverse Aging (HGH)	$10.00	$7.00
√D006	This Land Is Leached Land	$10.00	$7.00
√D007	Take it Off, Keep it Off	$10.00	$7.00
√D008	Undoing of Disease	$10.00	$7.00
√D009	Live Long and Prosper	$10.00	$7.00
√D012	Mineral Story	$10.00	$7.00
√D013	Y Factor	$10.00	$7.00
√D014	Dead Doctors Don't Lie	$10.00	$7.00
√D015	Mineral Basics	$10.00	$7.00
√D016	Health Confidence	$25.00	$14.00
	(Creflo Dollar's Church)		

LISTEN TO DR.WALLACH'S RADIO SHOW

Talk to Dr.Wallach live on Weekdays on
his Radio Programs:

"Dead Doctors Don't Lie"
Toll free   888-379-2552
Priority line: 831-685-1080
Live 12:00 noon - 1:00 pm Pacific Time

"Let's Play Doctor"
Toll free: 877-912-7529
Live 1:00 pm - 2:00 pm Pacific Time

Listen to Dr.Wallach's radio show on line
www.kscoradio.com
click on: "pod cast"
click on: "Dead Doctors Don't Lie"